ALTERNATIVES FOR EVERYONE

A Guide to Non-Traditional Health Care

Other books by Lauren O. Thyme:

Thymely Tales, Transformational Fairy Tales for Adults and Children, 2nd edition

The Lemurian Way: Remembering Your Essential Nature, 2nd edition (with Sareya Orion)

Forgiveness Equals Fortune (co-authored with Liah Holtzman), 2nd edition

Along the Nile, 2nd edition

From the Depths of Thyme

Strangers in Paradise, a novel of forgiveness

Cosmic Grandma Wisdom

Twin Souls, A Karmic Love Story

Traveling on the River of Time, a handbook for exploring past lives

Catherine, Karma and Complex PTSD (to be published in 2018)

ALTERNATIVES FOR EVERYONE

A Guide to Non-Traditional Health Care

Lauren O. Thyme

Lauren O. Thyme Publishing
Santa Fe, New Mexico
2017

Jacket/cover design:
Cover photo Pixabay flower-204161_960_72
Cover and interior design by Sue Stein

Special thanks to Sue Stein and Roy Briggs for their enormous help in creating this 2nd edition.

This book is dedicated in gratitude to my holistic physician,
Dr. Michael Kwiker, who told me in 1977,
"Wow! You are really sick!" and the rest is history.

Contents

HOLISTIC, PREVENTATIVE, AND ALTERNATIVE MEDICINE   17

HEALTH PRODUCTS

INTRODUCTION

My reason for creating this book is intensely personal. For most of my life I'd been sickly and unhappy, which kept me out of school and being able to play, hardly able to be satisfactorily employed nor healthfully parent my children. I received traditional medical care for years without much difference.

In 1974, immediately after giving birth to my second child, I became extremely ill and bedridden. Although I was only 27 years old, I felt like I was an ancient old woman.

I was alternately hungry or bloated, with constant stomach pain and indigestion. I was having difficulty breathing, along with many other physical symptoms. I was depressed, anxious, lacking in energy and vitality. I started having panic attacks and was diagnosed as agoraphobic. At one point I counted 40 symptoms ranging from physical to mental to emotional, which disturbed my job, my family, my outlook on life, my relationships, and my happiness.

What followed was a stream of specialists, internists, and psychotherapists as my family doctor couldn't figure out was wrong with me. I was treated with massive doses of antibiotics to treat an unknown bacteria. That medical treatment led to a vaginal infection I couldn't get rid of for 5 years. One diagnosis pointed to a pre-ulcer condition, so I was treated with medicine, antacids, and a bland diet. Another was that I was anxious, for which valium and therapy were prescribed.

I began sleeping 15-18 hours a day. I was hardly able to work. My stomach was upset and painful even with all the prescriptions I was taking. I didn't feel any better with drugs or therapy either. In fact, I felt worse. After a while I was afraid to go to work, shop, movies, drive, or even out into the back yard because of the panic attacks I was suffering. Life wasn't worth living. I was at the end of my emotional rope.

I read about hypoglycemia and asked an internist to perform a three-hour test of my blood sugar. He agreed, but afterwards told me my test results were odd but were nothing to worry about. Then he berated me for wasting his time and the insurance money. "It's patients like you who drive up the cost of health insurance." Maybe the doctor was right, that I was a hypochondriac.

Later I found out that my test results were classic for hypoglycemia.

My family and I relocated to Sacramento, thinking that the clearer air might help my breathing problems. When we settled in, I decided to try a new approach. The yellow pages advertised Sacramento Holistic and Preventative Medical Clinic, created by Dr. Garry Gordon. I made an appointment to see his associate, Dr. Michael Kwiker. What did I have to lose?

Before my initial visit, I filled out an in-depth four-page questionnaire of my symptoms and history. Then I had a 2 hour consultation with Dr. Kwiker. After questioning me thoroughly, he commented, "Wow! You are really sick!" I was 32 years old.

I broke down and cried. Finally, someone was listening.

The clinic ran a number of non-invasive tests. The resulting diagnoses was lengthy, which determined that I had hypoglycemia, thyroid and adrenal gland dysfunction, prolapsed colon, multiple food sensitivities, lack of hydrochloric acid necessary in digesting food, low to non-existent levels of vitamins and minerals, a hiatal hernia, and a few other problems.

A new world opened up for me. A special diet was prescribed, along with many vitamins, minerals, and herbs. I took hydrochloric acid for two years until I was finally able to digest proteins on my own. I also took glandular products to help my thyroid and adrenal glands. One of the special treatments was a weekly shot of adrenal cortex extract with massive amounts of vitamin C vitamin and B complex. The clinic had a non-force chiropractor on staff, whose efforts reduced my physical pain and helped heal the hiatal hernia. In the beginning I visited the clinic twice a week for various treatments, tests, and follow-ups. By the end of 5 years I was seeing them on an as-needed basis.

Although this clinic primarily treated me for physical problems, my doctor also recommended conscious breathing (rebirthing as it was called then). My poor self-esteem had led to a variety of emotional and psychological problems, which began to improve using this technique. I had over 100 sessions.

Impressed and eager, I began to search on my own for other alternative methods that might help my health improve even more. I investigated bodyworkers, psychotherapists, hypnotists, spiritual healers, nutritionists, and homeopaths, to name just a few. Most of the methods discussed in this book I have personally experienced and thus became quite knowledgeable.

Like my holistic doctor, these alternative health care practitioners listened carefully to what I said about my body, rather than insulted me, or told me there was nothing wrong. If I had symptoms and pain, then a problem obviously existed. And as long as there was a problem, they would continue to assist me.

My overall health improved. I realized that health would be a life-long process.

I was hired as Executive Director of the Sacramento Holistic Health Institute which, among other benefits, had a referral service to local alternative health care practitioners. Every week I hosted the guest lecture evenings. I read, studied, and took classes while I continued to schedule many forms of alternative health care treatment.

I realize I may have painted a bleak picture in regards to traditional medicine. I don't mean to insult that institution. However, I discovered that traditional medicine has limitations. What I envisioned in 1988 when I first published this book was that traditional and alternative medicine could work together hand in hand. Now in 2017 I witness marvelous shifts in the health care culture and am encouraged that miracles are on the horizon.

Thus this book is a labor of love. I have tried most of the techniques described herein. But Alternatives for Everyone is not simply about my own struggle and success. I'm sharing what I've learned in order to pass on valuable information to you.

Since the first edition of Alternatives for Everyone came out I have spoken with scores of people who were desperately looking for solutions to their struggles. I encouraged them to try alternative health care. I lectured in the community and to health care professionals.

If you are sick, in pain or suffering, but can't seem to get better, don't give up. Keep looking. There is a world of alternative health care to explore. If you have problems, there is an underlying cause—and perhaps a cure as well.

Alternatives for everyone exist today in ever-growing numbers and burgeoning information than when I first offered this book in 1988. I'm also including cutting-edge health care and products, although they may not be strictly classified as non-traditional.

In 1985–86 researching was a long-term, tedious chore. However now, because of the instant benefit of the internet, one can type in a word and a plethora of books, descriptions, and health care practitioners pop up almost instantly for review. My job, as I see it, is to gather all the methods I know into one volume to assist in your search, to give you a starting place. This book makes a great gift, too.

I consider health a verb, a journey, and a process, rather than a destination. In that regard health is ever-expanding. One can never have too much health.

One particular guide, which health food stores find indispensable, and often have a reference copy for customers, is listed below. An online look inside at the massive Amazon internet bookstore will take you to an index of this book where you can cross reference ailments and remedies quickly and easily.

A world of understanding and healing lies poised at your fingertips.

A votre sante! (to your health)
Lauren O. Thyme 2017

The Encyclopedia of Natural Medicine Third Edition by Michael T. Murray, Joseph Pizzorno; Simon and Schuster, NY, NY, 2012

DISCLAIMER

The purpose of this guide is to educate, inform, and even entertain. The author and publisher shall have neither liability nor responsibility to any person or entity with respect to any loss or damage caused or alleged to be caused directly or indirectly by the information contained in this book.

Alternatives for Everyone is designed to provide information in regard to the subject matter covered. The book is sold with the understanding that the publisher and author are not engaged in rendering medical, psychological, or other professional services. If medical or other expert assistance is required, the services of a competent professional should be sought. I, the author, am not medically trained to answer your questions, nor is the intention of this book to give medical advice.

I do not endorse nor sponsor any therapy, treatment, book, service or product listed in this book. Although I have undertaken most of the practices in *Alternatives for Everyone*, I have not personally investigated all of them. Please use your own discretion.

I have no knowledge of going rates, fees, or appropriate amounts to pay for treatments.

I am not responsible for any treatment you receive as a result of reading this book, or any consequences thereof, from using any methods listed. I am not responsible for consequences of non-traditional health care when emergency, urgent care, or any other health care was needed instead.

Any difficulty encountered must be dealt with on your own. I am not a legal advisor.

The possibility exists that what was accurate when I published this book is no longer accurate when you read it. Also possible is that the way you interpret a statement may not be how I meant it.

Every effort has been made to make this guide as complete and accurate as possible. Even though I have thoroughly checked my manuscript, there may be mistakes, both in editing and in content. Therefore, this text should be used only as a general guide and not as the ultimate source of alternative health care information.

HOW TO CHOOSE AND USE
AN ALTERNATIVE HEALTH
CARE PRACTITIONER

Alternative health care is similar to traditional health care in that you choose and hire the professional who treats you. I definitely believe in "shopping around" for a practitioner who meets my requirements. If that practitioner does not meet my expectations, then I feel comfortable in moving on to someone else instead.

This is your body and you get to decide who you will work with. You are your own advocate. Doctors work for you, not the other way around. They are, after all, still practicing.

How to begin or when you move to a new area

The hardest part of finding someone who practices the alternative health method that you are interested in is where to start. The same is true whether you are beginning your search, wanting to undertake a new method that interests you, or if you have moved to a new locale. If you are having difficulty locating an alternative health practitioner, method, or product, the following resources may be helpful:

- a local health food store, health food restaurant, and/or metaphysical book store who have periodicals, advertisements, and/or business cards from health practitioners, and the owner, manager, or employees that work there;
- the internet, to find a listing of practitioners in your area;
- a local chiropractor or acupuncturist who may be aware of other al-

ternative health practitioners in their area and may themselves practice some additional forms of healing;

- a New Thought Church such as Center for Conscious Living, Self-Realization Fellowship, Unity, and Unitarian Universalist, having local periodicals and advertisements, with pastors or members who know practitioners in your area;
- a health practitioner who practices the method you are interested in who lives in another area.

The main thing is to keep looking. Even though the method you are interested in may not be advertised as clearly as your neighborhood grocery store, it may be available with exploration on your part. A little digging can reveal treasures. Alternative health practitioners in general are particularly interested in lending a hand, giving information, and being supportive. When they find you are open-minded and interested in alternatives, they tend to be candid and giving.

Once you have found someone, then what?
Serious diseases and illnesses

All the therapies presented in this book have merit. However, if you are seriously ill and have not yet been diagnosed, picking a therapy might be difficult. Pivotal to your well-being is determining the problems you face and then working towards the solution. If you are not sure what your problem is, getting your problem diagnosed first is reasonable.

However, many alternative health practitioners are not trained to diagnose. Preventive and holistic practitioners and naturopathic doctors are trained to do so and have non-invasive tests they can perform.

Research

Once you know what your problem(s) is, you can then research what is known about various methods as to therapeutic effectiveness. An approach or combination of approaches that are effective on your problem would be wise. Often diseases and illnesses may require a variety of therapeutic methods in order to facilitate healing. For example, meditation has been used as part of alternative cancer treatment and has been found to be of great value. However, common sense dictates that if you have been diagnosed with cancer, you may wish to explore a number of other methods in addition to meditation.

Can you practice any methods on your own?

Methods that provide you with personal skills can be valuable. I am cost-conscious and found that alternative treatments can run into great expense. Many alternative health care methods are not yet covered by insurance or Medicare. However, there are systems you can learn, then use on your own at home, in your own time and space, for free. Yoga, t'ai chi, aerobics, nutrition, affirmations, conscious breathing, meditation, live foods and fasting are but a few examples of techniques that you can do on your own.

Combining traditional with alternative

If you wish to continue using traditional (also known as allopathic medicine), you may want to keep in mind:

- Your traditional doctor needs to know what alternative health care methods you are using.
- Your alternative health practitioner needs to know your current diagnosis, treatment and/or medication.
- Your traditional physician may be skeptical, wary, or even suggest you discontinue your alternative health care. The doctor may not understand the treatment you are receiving and be apprehensive for your well-being. I speak frankly to my traditional doctors and tell them what I am doing and what I intend to achieve. Sometimes they are doubtful. When I achieve success in alternative methods, I share the success with my doctor, who often begins to appreciate those methods. I believe I am educating my doctor who can then help other patients as well.
- You may feel that traditional and alternative health care do not blend well and you may experience frustration and confusion.
- Traditional and alternative health care may seem contradictory and conflicting to you.
- You may have to take your prescriptions for a while or even permanently, while you also take natural remedies such as homeopathy or herbs.

For example, I took a drug for a minor heart valve dysfunction. I worked on other areas of my health using alternative methods. After a year or so I was able to discontinue the drug altogether. I also had severe PMS and was taking the hormone progesterone, but it didn't help alleviate the symptoms. Then a homoeopathist prescribed a remedy. Within two months I was able to stop the hormone. The condition went away. I continued to successfully take the homeopathic remedy until I reached menopause, many years later.

Practice healthy skepticism

No individual practitioner or method is known to cure all forms of illness, pain, or disease for every patient. Keep an open mind yet allow your considerations and doubts to surface.

Be wary of any approach that says it is the only way to solve your problem.

I believe it is time to eliminate professional differences, both within the alternative field itself and between traditional and alternative health. Each has value to share with us and each has its limitations. I wouldn't dream of discarding traditional medicine.

However, alternative health offers assistance where traditional medicine is just beginning to venture, into the subtleties of health, the complexities of bodies and minds, beyond Western scientific thought and research, into preventive care, and remedies both ancient and modern. My dream is for us to see into the future where traditional and alternative health care work side by side for the benefit of us all.

Therefore, I think it is wise to avoid practitioners who want to exclude other potentially beneficial treatments.

Methods that work great for you may not work well for other people. Methods that work great for other people may not be beneficial for you. Since we are all unique, each person's path to wellness is going to be individual, differing from the other billions of souls living on this planet in chemical make-up, personality, background, genes, wants, desires, and an indefinable something called "spirit."

I advise you carefully research any method or practitioner that a friend or acquaintance raves about. If you "just can't miss it," maybe you had better.

Check out testimonials and trust yourself. Some of the worst practices and practitioners I have experienced were based on friends' advice. I love my friends—but—I have to find my own remedies and thoroughly vet a practitioner.

Is the cure worse than the problem?

Evaluate the potential harm of a treatment. This is true of both traditional and alternative health care.

- Will your body be invaded by treatment or by a diagnostic tool?
- Are there side-effects to the treatments? If so, what?
- Are the remedies toxic or do they work in harmony with the body? Are they from natural sources or created in a laboratory? Might you experience an allergic reaction? For example, some herbs can be toxic if taken every day.
- Are substitutions available and are they as effective?

Be a health care detective

Examine and evaluate the practitioner's credentials, background, training and integrity.

What certification does the health practitioner have – MD, DO, DC, ND, CMT, CA, etc? You might want to find out what the initials stand for and what it represents in terms of training and education.

Does the practitioner belong to an association or organization which promotes their method(s)?

Find out the practitioner's viewpoint concerning their on-going education. Many reputable practitioners are interested in continuing to educate themselves, not only in the areas they practice, but in other alternative fields as well.

Be aware of extraordinary claims or vague explanations.

Alternative health care practitioners are trained in ways and use methods that are often unfamiliar to most people and traditional medical providers. This training may be in "non-scientific" or non-Western ways of thinking. Because of that people, and traditional medicine as well, have mistrusted, feared, and were unsure about alternative health care, calling them quacks and cults with dubious and false claims. Who can you believe? To evaluate a potential practitioner by determining details of training, claims, and concrete evidence is to assist you in finding quality practitioners.

Beware of someone who calls him or herself "doctor" but who has no medical degree nor a degree that's comparable from a recognized school. Naturopaths are doctors as are chiropractors and dentists.

Usually payment is due upon treatment. Beware of therapies that you sign up for and pay for in advance. I would be suspicious of someone wanting me to pay for a treatment that I hadn't yet received. Find out why the therapy must be paid for in advance. Are there discounts involved for multiple treatments? I would want to wait until I had experienced that practitioner (and method) before contracting for future sessions, no matter the discount.

Evaluate

You may want to evaluate the practitioner in relationship to his/her health care method. You can call or email the organization or association that represents the method you are researching. You can find out if your particular practitioner needs to be licensed, certified, or needing membership in that organization in order to be recognized and approved to practice.

Does that practitioner need to be trained and educated at their approved facility in order to be called that kind of practitioner? If so, was your practitioner trained there? Trager, Rolfing, and Touch for Health are but a few who require training at an approved facility or by a certified trainer.

Talk to Others

You can ask your potential practitioner if he/she has any clients with whom you can speak. Talk to others who have consulted with or been treated by that practitioner. Talk to two or three people if possible and keep an open mind. I recommend avoiding being either too gullible or too skeptical.

You can also talk to other people who have experienced the method you are considering.

Multi-Faceted

Does your prospective practitioner have some knowledge about both traditional and alternative health care? Those who have more in-depth knowledge about traditional health care have usually schooled themselves intensely, or are former traditional health caretakers who have gone seeking for something more.

In contrast be cautious of someone who is insistent on avoiding traditional medical care. Simply because traditional health care has limitations does not diminish its value and importance in our society. I am wary of practitioners who wants to "throw the baby out with the bathwater."

Communicate. Communicate. Communicate.

If possible, interview your practitioner before you decide to begin treatment or diagnostics. Seeing, hearing, and sensing this person in the flesh can be illuminating. The practitioner may sound great on the phone or have a wonderful resume on the internet but you may feel uncomfortable with him or her in person. Trust your gut instincts. This is your body and your emotions (and your hard-earned money) that you are delegating to this person.

A practitioner needs to have a caring, humane approach and be a person with whom you can discuss the personal details of your life. Besides being competent and well-trained, being caring is one of the single most important elements of your practitioner. I have noticed that the practitioners who "cared" about me are the ones with whom I experienced the most healing, transformation, and change.

I believe this caring comes from a personal interest. Many times, people who have either created an alternative health care method or those who practice the method have often used it to heal themselves or a loved one first. When the results were inspiring, these people went on to share it with others who were suffering. I call this "heart motivation." Just as my heart motivated me to share the information in this book with you.

Feeling compatible with your practitioner and his/her practice is vitally significant. For me there is nothing more uncomfortable than to be with a practitioner (who otherwise is well trained, reputable, listens well, etc.) but his or her beliefs, office environment, personality, and other factors may interfere with a working relationship. The two of you are a team.

Beware that your desire and desperation—or even fear—to get well, may make you overlook your instincts and feelings regarding a practitioner or a method because you want to get healthy. Just because it helped someone else doesn't mean it will help you. Pay attention.

Communicate some more

Communication is vital. Be sure to discuss any questions, fears, concerns, symptoms, discomfort, problems, side effects, pain, improvement, or anything that feels "funny" to you. Mention everything. Nothing is insignificant. If need be, keep a list and bring it to consultations and treatments. If your complaints worsen, call your practitioner. During treatment, communicate as well, particularly during bodywork or psychological therapy.

Trust what your body and your intuition tells you

You are the final word on your health. You are the expert on yourself and have lived with yourself for decades. You have a Ph.D. on "you."

Pain in your body is real, regardless of the cause. A reason exists for aches, pains, and symptoms. Those are your body's way of communicating with you regarding any imbalances in your body, mind, and emotions. In alternative medicine the cause of many of those imbalances can be determined and a solution brought about.

Consequently, I don't believe in the definition of "hypochondriac." Instead there exist suffering human beings who have not yet found the right path to wellness, whether that path is physical, mental, emotional, spiritual or a combination of those. If you don't feel good, a reason exists. Your job is to keep looking. Alternative health care practitioners are members of your personal team to help find the cause and a solution.

Dis-ease (or lack of ease) on one level affects the other levels of your entire being.

You do not need to experience pain while in treatment. "No pain, no gain," is not a necessary maxim to good health. This is particularly true of bodywork. If you are experiencing pain during a session, tell your bodyworker. Sometimes pain is stored and comes to the surface during a session. You are in charge. If the pain or discomfort is more than you want or can handle, let your bodyworker know as it is happening.

What to do in an emergency

Alternative health care practitioners may not respond to emergencies and urgent care. Generally, alternative practitioners are for on-going and preventive care. Many, or most, have not been trained in emergent or urgent care. Having a back-up health care system for that possibility is a good idea. If need be, you can find a traditional health care doctor who can serve in emergencies or you can go to an urgent care facility or hospital emergency room. If you do get urgent or emergency care, be sure to let your alternative health care practitioner know the details.

Are you getting results?

If you are not achieving the results you want, discuss this with your practitioner.

Progress may seem too slow, but alternative health care takes more time than traditional medicine. Your body is healing from the inside out and drugs are not masking symptoms. As you become more sensitive to your body, you may notice results more clearly.

You may get worse before you get better. This is known as the "healing crisis" and nothing to be alarmed about. Your body is stepping in to activate its complex innate healing mechanisms.

For example, the usual way to treat a cold is to go to the medicine cabinet or drug store, and take a cold remedy or aspirin. In alternative medicine, many believe a cold is the body's way of removing toxins which are interfering with the proper function of the body. Mucus accumulated through improper diet may build up and then begin to drip. A fever may result, which means the body is burning off toxins. The body perspires to remove impurities through the pores. We get tired, which is the body telling us to rest while it heals itself. We get thirsty as the body wants to wash itself with liquids to aid in the cleansing process. While we seem sick, we are actually in a healing crisis; we are improving.

Alternative health care takes time and patience. You may be disappointed if you are expecting instant results or an instant cure. Give yourself, your body, and your practitioner adequate time to achieve improved health. If, after discussion, more work, and sufficient time has elapsed, you are still not satisfied, you may decide to move on to a new practitioner or a different method.

Good fortune to you in your search for improved health.

Alternative Medicine: The Definitive Guide (2nd Edition); John W. Anderson (Editor), Larry Trivieri (Editor), 2002, Celestial Arts, NY, NY

HOLISTIC, PREVENTATIVE, AND ALTERNATIVE MEDICINE

Holistic medicine is a form of healing that considers the whole person — body, mind, spirit, and emotions—in the quest for optimal health and wellness. According to the holistic medicine philosophy, one can achieve optimal health—the primary goal of holistic medicine practice—by gaining proper balance in life. Holistic medicine practitioners believe that the whole person is made up of interdependent parts and if one part is not working properly, all the other parts will be affected. If people have physical, emotional, or spiritual imbalances in their lives, it can negatively affect their overall health.

A holistic doctor may use all forms of health care, from conventional medication to alternative therapies, to treat a patient. For example, when a person suffering from migraine headaches pays a visit to a holistic doctor, instead of walking out solely with medications, the doctor will likely take a look at all the potential factors that may be causing the person's headaches, such as other health problems, diet and sleep habits, stress and personal problems, and preferred spiritual practices. The treatment plan involves supplements, but also lifestyle modifications to help prevent the headaches from recurring.

Holistic medicine is also based on the belief that a person is ultimately responsible for his or her own health and well-being. Other principles of holistic medicine include the following:

- All people have innate healing powers;
- The patient is a person, not a disease;
- Healing takes a team approach involving both the patient and doctor,

and addresses all aspects of a person's life using a variety of health care practices;

- Treatment involves fixing the cause of the condition, not just alleviating the symptoms.

Holistic practitioners use a variety of treatment techniques to aid their patients to take responsibility for their own well-being and achieve optimal health. Depending on the practitioner's training, these may include:

- Patient education on lifestyle changes and self-care to promote wellness. This may include diet, exercise, psychotherapy, relationship and spiritual counseling, and more;
- Complementary and alternative therapies such as acupuncture, chiropractic care, homeopathy, massage therapy, naturopathy, supplements, and others;
- Western medications and surgical procedures.

Preventive healthcare consists of measures taken for disease prevention, as opposed to disease treatment. Just as health encompasses a variety of physical and mental states, so do disease and disability, which are affected by environmental factors, genetic predisposition, disease agents, and lifestyle choices. Ill health, disease, and disability are dynamic processes which begin before individuals realize they are affected. Disease prevention relies on actions that can be categorized as primal, primary, secondary, and tertiary prevention.

Each year, millions of people die of preventable deaths. A 2004 study showed that about half of all deaths in the United States in 2000 were due to preventable behaviors and exposures.

Leading causes included cardiovascular disease, chronic respiratory disease, unintentional injuries, diabetes, and certain infectious diseases. This same study estimates that 400,000 people die each year in the United States due to poor diet and a sedentary lifestyle. According to estimates made by the World Health Organization, about 55 million people died worldwide in 2011, 66% of this group from non-communicable diseases, including cancer, diabetes, and chronic cardiovascular and lung diseases. This is an increase from the year 2000, during which 60% of deaths were attributed to these diseases. Preventive healthcare is especially important given the worldwide rise in chronic diseases and deaths from these diseases.

There are many methods for prevention of disease. Adults and children are encouraged to visit their doctor for regular check-ups, even if they feel healthy, to perform disease screening, identify risk factors for disease, discuss tips for a healthy and balanced lifestyle, and maintain a good relationship with a healthcare provider.

Some common disease screenings include checking for high blood pressure; high blood sugar (a risk factor for diabetes mellitus); high blood cholesterol; screening for colon cancer; depression; HIV and other sexually transmitted diseases such as chlamydia, syphilis, and gonorrhea; mammography to screen for breast cancer; colorectal cancer screening; a pap test to check for cervical cancer; and x-ray screening for osteoporosis. Genetic testing can also be performed to screen for mutations that cause genetic disorders or predisposition to certain diseases such as breast or ovarian cancer.

Preventive medicine is practiced by all physicians to keep their patients healthy and is also a unique medical specialty recognized by the American Board of Medical Specialties (ABMS). Preventive medicine focuses on the health of individuals, communities, and defined populations, while its goal is to protect, promote, and maintain health and well-being and to prevent disease, disability, and death.

Preventive medicine specialists are licensed medical doctors (MD), doctors of osteopathy (DO), and naturopaths (ND), who possess core competencies in biostatistics, epidemiology, environmental and occupational medicine, planning and evaluation of health services, management of health care organizations, research into causes of disease and injury in population groups, and the practice of prevention in clinical medicine. They apply knowledge and skills gained from the medical, social, economic, and behavioral sciences.

Preventive medicine has three specialty areas with common core knowledge, skills, and competencies that emphasize different populations, environments, or practice settings: aerospace medicine; occupational medicine; and public health and general preventive medicine. ACPM members generally focus on public health and general preventive medicine, but many of the members are double or triple board-certified in multiple specialty areas.

AROMATHERAPY

Aromatherapy uses plant materials and aromatic plant oils, including essential oils, and other aroma compounds for improving psychological or physical well-being. It can be offered as a complementary therapy or, more controversially, as a form of alternative medicine.

Aromatherapists who specialize in the practice of aromatherapy utilize blends of therapeutic essential oils that can be delivered through topical application, massage, inhalation or water immersion to stimulate a desired response.

The use of essential oils for therapeutic, spiritual, hygienic, and ritualistic purposes goes back to ancient civilizations including the Chinese, Indians, Egyptians, Greeks, and Romans who used them in cosmetics, perfumes, and drugs.

Oils are described by Dioscorides, along with beliefs of the time regarding their healing properties, in his De Materia Medica, written in the first century. Distilled essential oils have been employed as medicines since the invention of distillation in the eleventh century, when Avicenna isolated essential oils using steam distillation.

The concept of aromatherapy was first introduced in 1907 by a small number of European scientists and doctors. In 1937, the word first appeared in print in a French book on the subject: Aromathérapie: Les Huiles Essentielles, Hormones Végétales by René-Maurice Gattefossé, a chemist. An English version of that book was published in 1993. In 1910, Gattefossé badly burned his hand and later claimed he treated it effectively with lavender oil.

A French surgeon, Jean Valnet, pioneered the medicinal uses of essential oils, which he used as antiseptics in the treatment of wounded soldiers during World War II.

The modes of application of aromatherapy include:
- Aerial diffusion: for environmental fragrance or aerial disinfection;
- Direct inhalation: for respiratory disinfection, decongestant, expectoration as well as psychological effects;

- Topical applications: for general massage, baths, compresses, therapeutic skin care.

Some of the materials include:

- Essential oils: fragrant oils extracted from plants chiefly through steam distillation (e.g., eucalyptus oil) or expression (grapefruit oil). However, the term is also occasionally used to describe fragrant oils extracted from plant material by solvent extraction. This material includes incense reed diffusers.
- Absolutes: fragrant oils extracted primarily from flowers or delicate plant tissues through solvent or supercritical fluid extraction (e.g., rose absolute). The term is also used to describe oils extracted from fragrant butters, and effleurage pomades using ethanol.
- Carrier oils: typically oily plant base triacylglycerides that dilute essential oils for use on the skin (e.g., sweet almond oil).
- Herbal distillates or hydrosols: the aqueous by-products of the distillation process (e.g., rosewater). Common herbal distillates are chamomile, rose, and lemon balm.
- Infusions: aqueous extracts of various plant material (e.g., infusion of chamomile).
- Phytoncides: various volatile organic compounds from plants that kill microbes. Many terpene-based fragrant oils and sulfuric compounds from plants in the genus Allium (e.g. onions and garlic) are phytoncides, though the latter are likely less commonly used in aromatherapy due to their disagreeable odors.
- Aroma lamp or diffuser: an electric or candle-fueled device which volatilizes essential oils, usually mixed with water.
- Vaporizer: typically higher oil content plant based materials dried, crushed, and heated to extract and inhale the aromatic oil vapors in a direct inhalation modality.

AYURVEDA

Ayurveda (Sanskrit: life-knowledge) or Ayurvedic medicine is a system of medicine with historical roots in the Indian subcontinent. Globalized and modernized practices derived from Ayurveda traditions are a type of complementary or alternative medicine. In the Western world, Ayurveda therapies and practices have been integrated into alternative health care and medical use.

The central theoretical ideas of Ayurveda developed in the mid-first millennium BCE and show parallels with Sāṅkhya, Vaiśeṣika, Buddhism, and Jainism philosophies. Balance is emphasized, and suppressing natural urges is considered unhealthy and claimed to lead to illness.

The classical Ayurveda texts begin with accounts of the transmission of medical knowledge from the gods to sages, and then to human physicians. Ayurveda therapies have varied and evolved over more than two millennia. Therapies are typically based on complex herbal compounds, minerals, and metal substances. Ancient Ayurveda texts also taught surgical techniques, including rhinoplasty, kidney stone removal, sutures, and the extraction of foreign objects.

In medieval classifications of the Sanskrit knowledge systems, Ayurveda is assigned a place as a subsidiary Veda. Some medicinal plant names from the Atharvaveda and other Vedas can be found in subsequent Ayurveda literature. The earliest recorded theoretical statements about the canonical models of disease in Ayurveda occur in the earliest Buddhist Canon.

Ayurveda names seven basic tissues: plasma, blood, muscles, fat, bone, marrow, and semen. Like the medicine of classical antiquity, Ayurveda has historically divided bodily substances into five classical elements: earth, water, fire, air and ether. There are also twenty gunas (qualities or characteristics) which are considered to be inherent in all substances. These are organized in ten pairs of antonyms: heavy/light, cold/hot, unctuous/dry, dull/sharp, stable/mobile, soft/hard, non-slimy/slimy, smooth/coarse, minute/gross, and viscous/liquid.

Ayurveda has eight ways to diagnose illness: pulse, urine, stool, tongue, speech, touch, vision, and appearance. Ayurvedic practitioners diagnose by using the five senses. For example, hearing is used to observe the condition of breathing and speech.

Ayurvedic doctors regard physical existence, mental existence, and personality as a unit, with each element able to influence the others. This is a holistic approach used during diagnosis and therapy, and is a fundamental aspect of Ayurveda. Another part of Ayurvedic treatment says there are channels which transport fluids, and that the channels can be opened up by massage treatment using oils and fomentation. Unhealthy channels are thought to cause disease.

BATES METHOD

The Bates method is a therapy aimed at improving eyesight. Eye-care physician William Horatio Bates, M.D. (1860–1931) attributed nearly all sight problems to habitual strain of the eyes, and felt that glasses were harmful and unnecessary. Bates self-published a book, *Perfect Sight Without Glasses*, as well as a magazine, "Better Eyesight Magazine," detailing his approach to helping people relax eye strain, and thus, he claimed, improving their sight. His techniques centered on visualization and movement.

He placed particular emphasis on imagining black letters and marks, and the movement of those. He also felt that exposing the eyes to sunlight would help alleviate the strain. An anecdotal report of successful results, including well-publicized support for the Bates method, was testified to by many, as well as the well-known author Aldous Huxley.

In addition to perceiving fine detail, eyes are constantly active and receptive to the visual world in many other respects. The eyes perceive light, darkness, shade, color, movement, form, and depth. These attributes, while important, are often taken for granted.

In contrast to this visual foundation, the modern and technological world pushes the eyes to become transmitters for information, taking us away from the natural uses of the eyes and mind that our ancestors enjoyed. The visual system is now used extensively to read and interpret the written word or process visual media, presenting the mind with abstract ideas with which to engage or make decisions; such as finishing a report, figuring out one's taxes, or reading a book. If a person has a tendency to eyestrain, these distractions can take on an addictive quality, with the natural state of the visual system a long forgotten memory.

Modern culture takes the eyes and mind out of the present and into a world where what the mind sees is not what the eyes see; the mind is busy creating abstractions, imaginings, stresses, and worries.

This is not to say that interpretation of the written word or the television screen is inherently at fault for the production of eyesight problems, but that the lack of pure and natural visual experience has become an issue of epidemic proportions. The greater the hold of the interpretational mind, the harder it becomes to simply enjoy seeing for what it is; so much so that it becomes clear that even when there is a pure visual scene in front of a person, the mind can still be far away thinking about other things.

All the Bates techniques simply require a person to look at colors, shapes, depths, textures, shades, and movements, all of which are nourishment for the eyes and in every waking moment, what the eyes see.

If the mind is closed to the world, busy with other things, all that visual information has nowhere to go, and eventually the eyes begin to suffer. But if you look at what is in front of you right now, you come fully into the present moment. Any avoidance of where and who you are right now evaporates.

The techniques taught in the Bates Method effectively re-establish the normal, natural interaction between eye and mind. To the visually-impaired person, perceiving movement, or letting the eyes feast on color can seem odd or contrived, but what is happening is that the mind is learning slowly how to dismantle its filters.

CANDIDA THERAPY

Every person lives in a virtual sea of microorganisms of bacteria, viruses, and fungi. These microbes reside in the throat, mouth, nose, and intestinal tract. They are as much a part of our bodies as the food we eat. Usually, these microorganisms do not cause illness, unless our resistance becomes lowered. Candida albicans is a yeast that lives in the mouth, throat, intestines and genitourinary tract of most humans and is usually considered to be a normal part of the bowel flora, the organisms that coexist with us in our lower digestive tract.

Candida enters newborn infants during or shortly after birth. Usually, the growth of the yeast is kept in check by the infant's immune system and produces no overt symptoms. But if the immune response weakens, the condition known as oral thrush can occur as a result. By six months of age,

90% of all babies test positive for Candida and by adulthood, virtually all humans play host to Candida albicans and are thus engaged in a life-long relationship.

Candida coexists in our bodies with many species of bacteria in a competitive balance. Other bacteria act in partnership to keep Candida growth in check in our body ecology, unless that balance is upset. The problem begins when the normal Candida species that we have in our gut changes form to disease-causing. This happens when the gut and other tissues becomes more acidic, either through taking a variety of drugs that wipe out the lactobacillus species, or through eating acidic foods. When health is present, the immune system keeps Candida proliferation under control, but when immune response is weakened, Candida growth can proceed unhindered. The uncontrolled growth of Candida is known as Candida overgrowth or Candidiasis.

- Contributors to Candida overgrowth:
- Steroid hormones and immunosuppressant drugs;
- Pregnancy, multiple pregnancies, or birth control pills;
- Diets high in carbohydrate and sugar intake, yeast and yeast products, as well as molds and fermented foods;
- Prolonged exposure to environmental molds;
- Antibiotics and sulfa drugs, including antibiotic-treated foods such as meats, dairy, poultry and eggs. Antibiotics kill all bacteria, the good with the bad.
- Menstruation;
- Sperm;
- Diabetes.

Symptoms of Candidiasis:
- feeling sluggish or exhausted, even after getting out of bed;
- recurring joint pain;
- recurring depression or experiencing a funk;
- irritable or anxious;
- foggy or hard to concentrate;
- digestive problems, chronic skin irritation, or migraines;

- a low libido;
- catching colds too easily or too often;
- unable to lose weight even after many diets;
- vaginal pain, swelling, and unpleasant discharge;
- mouth feels cottony and the sense of taste is impaired;
- cracking, swelling or bleeding skin;
- may be related to irritable bowel syndrome and neurological dysfunction.

Treatment:
- Plant-derived antifungal medication
- Antifungal diet, including steroid, hormone, and antibiotic-free food
- Probiotics

CHELATION THERAPY

Chelation therapy is a medical procedure that involves the administration of specific chelating agents to remove heavy metals from the body. Chelation therapy has a long history of use in clinical toxicology and remains in use for specific medical treatments.

Chelation therapy is the preferred medical treatment for metal poisoning, including acute mercury, iron, arsenic, lead, uranium, plutonium, and other forms of toxic metal poisoning. The chelating agent may be administered intravenously, intramuscularly, or orally, depending on the agent and the type of poisoning. Certain chelating drugs bind to heavy metals in the body and prevent them from binding to other agents, and are then excreted from the body.

Chelation is thought to help remove calcium build up known as plaque in the arteries; this method is still under discussion and scrutiny.

COLON HYDROTHERAPY;
COLON IRRIGATION; COLONICS

Colon hydrotherapy is the gentle rinsing of the colon with warm water, to remove encrusted fecal matter, gas, and mucus. This allows vital nutrients to be absorbed more easily and leaves the patient feeling rejuvenated and healthier. Colonics can also help re-tone and reshape the colon.

Colon hydrotherapy involves the safe, gentle infusion of water into the colon via the rectum. No chemicals or drugs are involved and the entire therapy is both relaxing and effective. A healthy well-functioning bowel is essential for the maintenance of optimal health. This vital organ remains the most neglected in the human body.

Because of modern diets full of animal proteins, processed food, fat, and sugar, along with stress and lack of exercise, the colon becomes the repository of accumulated waste and toxins which disable the body's purification system. The toxic material ends up re-entering our blood stream and getting deposited in our cells. When the blood stream is overloaded with toxic waste, the body will function at a lower level. As a result of this auto-intoxication we feel and act far below our potential and can become susceptible to disease.

Colon hydrotherapy is very safe when performed by a qualified therapist. FDA approved medical devices are used for the procedure and all of the equipment used is sterilized or disposable. The water goes through an advanced filtration process prior to entering the colon. ARCH (Association of Registered Colon Hydrotherapists) are trained and registered and meet the highest professional and ethical standards.

The benefits of colonics can include increased energy, improved circulation, clearer skin and eyes, mental clarity, weight normalizing, better digestion, and relief from bloating and heaviness. By removing the waste material from the colon, the process of detoxification is given a boost and the harmful bacteria produced by encrusted fecal matter is removed from the body. Colon hydrotherapy helps your immune system to help itself, by giving it a chance to breathe and allow the lymph system to effectively cleanse your body.

Colon hydrotherapy can assist the body with healing a variety of conditions: constipation, diarrhea, irritable bowel, bloating, excessive gas, indigestion, allergies, candida overgrowth, skin problems, brittle nails and hair, abnormal body odor, unpleasant breath, backache, stiffness, arthritis, fatigue, insomnia, poor concentration, and headaches.

ENVIRONMENTAL MEDICINE; MULTIPLE CHEMICAL SENSITIVITIES

Multiple chemical sensitivity (MCS) has been described under various names since the 1940s. MCS is a syndrome in which multiple symptoms occur with environmental exposure. The cause of MCS includes allergies, molds, pollens, dust, and neuro-biologic sensitization from many different chemicals and smells.

Environmental factors in the causation of environmental diseases can be classified into:

- Physical
- Chemical—the term chemical is used to refer broadly to many man-made chemical agents, some of which have multiple chemical constituents.
- Biological
- Social (including psychological and culture variables)
- Ergonomic
- Safety
- Any combination of the above

People are exposed to multiple chemicals every day at stores, businesses, and in our homes. This includes fluoride in drinking water and dental products, perfumes, scented products, carpeting, paints, fertilizers, pesticides, gardening supplies, cleaning items, vaccines, toiletries, shampoos, hair rinse, beauty supplies, and makeup. Harmful chemicals from our homes and businesses and toxins from everyday products as well as in our food has led to the increase of environmental illness.

Patients with MCS experience problems with depression, anxiety, chronic fatigue, fibromyalgia, autoimmune disorders such as rheumatoid arthritis and systemic lupus, cancer, and adult-onset diabetes. Often patients feel the need for extensive withdrawal from the outside world in order to heal.

Environmental medicine is a multidisciplinary field involving medicine, environmental science, chemistry and others, overlapping with environmental pathology. It may be viewed as the medical branch of the broader field of environmental health. The scope of this field involves studying the interactions between environment and human health, and the role of the environment in causing or mediating disease. In the United States, the American College of Occupational and Environmental Medicine (OCOEM) oversees board certification of physicians in environmental and occupational medicine. This board certification is recognized by the American Board of Medical Specialties.

There is a treatment option for patients—LDA—an antigen substance which can be homeopathic and/or injectable, after patients first being thoroughly tested for specific allergens. Healing measures also include exclusively using non-toxic, unscented products in all areas of life.

FASTING

Some people are afraid of fasting because they believe it is dangerous or detrimental to their well-being or they will feel deprived. To fast is to abstain from food while one possesses adequate reserves to nourish vital tissues, whereas to starve is to abstain from food after reserves have been exhausted so that vital tissues are sacrificed. Therefore, fasting is a simple, quick, powerful way to cleanse the body without starving and to help the healing process from illness and disease.

During fasting no food at all is taken but liquids are given in copious amounts. Those liquids can include delicious raw juices of fruits and vegetables, preferably fresh, as juices lose much of their valuable vitamins, minerals, trace elements, and enzymes within minutes of juicing. Vitamin-rich vegetable broths can be consumed as well as herbal teas.

Benefits to fasting:
- The body will live on itself, will burn and digest its own tissues after three days starting with those which are diseased, damaged, aged, or dead.
- The building of new healthy cells is speeded up.
- The capacity of lung, liver, kidneys, and skin is greatly increased, while masses of wastes and toxins are eliminated.
- Allows digestive, assimilative, and protective organs to rest and regenerate.
- Fasting exerts normalizing, stabilizing, and restorative effects on vital physiological, nervous, and mental functions.

- Fasting is beneficial in acute and in chronic disease. Colds, bronchitis, tonsillitis, as well as rheumatoid arthritis, asthma, diverticulitis, gout, constipation, and kidney problems benefit from fasting. Weight loss can be a byproduct of fasting and some weight loss programs use it to reduce obesity.
- Fasting can be used as a general health measure. Many sources advise to fast regularly, to keep the body clean. Fasting may help to overcome addictions to coffee, tea, smoking, and alcohol as well as to refined carbohydrates.
- Fasting can be done for one meal a day, for one day, for many days at a time, or for an extended duration under a doctor's care.

FLOWER ESSENCES

Dr. Richard Bach was both a traditional physician as well as a homeopathic doctor. He left London and his practice in 1930 to restore his health. He sought health in the healing benefits of flowers, using the same techniques as in homeopathy.

The system of flower essence therapeutics was originally used in ancient times, then revived by Dr. Bach who used English-derived flower essences. Bach prepared essences of 38 different flowers, each responding to a personality imbalance, and awakening the dormant inner quality to replace that imbalance. He believed, as do researchers of today, that fixed personality patterns have physical consequences. Types tend toward particular diseases (e.g., Type A personalities tend toward heart disease). His theory is that disease can arise from fears, anxieties, or likes and dislikes. The flower remedies work, not by attacking the disease, but by flooding the body with the vibrations of a higher nature. Bach believed that there can be no true healing unless there is a change in outlook, peace of mind, and inner happiness.

Dr. Bach saw three steps in the healing cycle using flower essences:
- A person must become aware of the personality pattern.
- A person must take responsibility for having created the present state of health.
- A person then takes the appropriate flower essences, transforming and healing the personality pattern.

Sometimes while healing habitual emotional patterns, a person may experience an upsetting healing crisis. But flower remedies are health catalysts which energize the health process without unduly interfering in its natural flow.

Since Dr. Bach's death, flower remedies from other countries have been available to treat an expanded repertory of emotional states.

FOOD COMBINING

Food combining deflates the theory of the four basic food groups in nutrition. When certain foods combine with each other properly it will enhance health, create more energy, and help a person feel great. But if foods are combined improperly then weight gain, loss of energy, even disease can result.

Food combining is based on the discovery that certain combinations of foods may be digested with greater ease and efficiency than others. There are 700 types of digestive enzymes for different foods. If these do not combine well, indigestion results. When food is properly combined and eaten, the digestive process is made easy, and energy is opened up for other uses.

The digestion of food demands more energy than any other human function. Digestion is divided into three cycles and includes digestion, assimilation of nutrients into the cells, and elimination— removing toxic wastes from the body. Digestion goes on 24 hours a day through these three cycles. If energy is needed for use elsewhere, this energy comes from the digestive tract.

One of the first people who studied food combining was Ivan Pavlov, famous for his experiments with dogs. In 1902 he published a book entitled The Work of the Digestive Glands where he revealed the basic fundamentals of proper food combining. Since then this subject has been the object of ongoing study and research. The main idea behind food combining is that the human body is not designed to digest more than one concentrated food in the stomach at the same time. Any food which is not a fruit nor a vegetable is concentrated. Carbohydrates and proteins are then classified as concentrated foods.

To eat a number of concentrated foods at the same time, such as a meat or cheese sandwich, pasta with cheese, pasta with sauce, meat and potatoes, cereal and milk, bacon/egg/toast/potatoes or any meal with fruit places a tremendous burden on the digestive system, creates toxicity in the body, and wastes vital energy.

When protein and carbohydrates are consumed together, the food is never properly digested. The stomach keeps pouring out hydrochloric acid which is neutralized by other enzymes. After a few hours the food is moved out of the stomach where it putrefies in the intestines. Nutrients cannot be utilized when fermentation and putrefaction occur and the body cannot build healthy cells. Instead of resolving the problem, many people medicate with antacids, laxatives, and prescription drugs which complicates the problem.

Food that is meant to digest in 30 minutes to 3 hours may stay in the stomach for up to 8 hours. Instead of passing through the intestines in 12 hours, improperly combined food may rot there instead for as long as 40 hours. After a lifetime of eating this way, tiredness, over-acidity, and over-weight is the result. The body is taxed beyond what it has been designed to cope with. Toxic waste builds up and certain body parts may begin to break down—which may cause diabetes, cancer, and other ailments.

Proper combining options are steak with salad and other vegetables, or pasta with stir-fry. The list is endless. Food combining also goes well with eating live foods and high-water content foods. Therefore food combining recommends eating raw foods and freshly-squeezed appropriate juices that are high in nutrients and water.

Food combining can relieve digestive problems such as; acid indigestion; ulcers; gas; heartburn; constipation; abdominal pain, sleeplessness; food allergies and sensitivities; and foul stools.

FOOD ROTATION AND DETOXIFICATION

A person may become sensitive or allergic to certain foods especially if that food is eaten regularly, every day, many times a day, or more often than every four days. Food allergies or sensitivities tax the immune system, trigger cravings of the very foods that are the problem, while causing the body to retain and increase weight in the form of fat. Continuing to eat those foods cause a person to be on a downward spiral towards illness, fatigue, psychological complaints, chronic disease, and more weight. Sensitivities and allergies cause toxic reactions in the body, causing cerebral problems, irritations, and serious illness.

Food sensitivity symptoms:

- **Chest and stomach**—fullness in chest, asthma, congestion or fluid in the lungs, persistent coughs, hoarseness, palpitations, rapid heart rate, vomiting, gas and flatulence, diarrhea, constipation, stomach feels heavy and bloated long after meals;
- **Psychological problems**—confusion, lethargy, aggression, irritability, hyperactivity, anxiety, depression, crying easily, inability to concentrate, trouble sleeping, sudden sleepiness soon after meals, and loss of sex drive;
- **Skin problems**—red spots, rashes, dermatitis, eczema, hives, and itching;
- **Extremities**—weakness in limbs, sore muscles, muscular aches and pains, joint pains, swelling of legs, feet, ankles and hands;
- **Miscellaneous symptoms**—chronic fatigue, urgency of urination, excessive hunger, rapid or significant changes in weight.

Food testing is recommended. If after testing, a person is determined to have one or more food sensitivities or allergies, then a food rotation diet is begun:

- Each food is eliminated from the diet, generally for two months;
- Each food is reintroduced systematically back into the diet one at a time;
- Each food is not to be eaten more than every four days.

A food diary is kept to note any reactions. A particular food may need to be permanently eliminated from the diet. Foods that often lead to sensitivities because they are staples in Western diets and also may be genetically modified are: wheat; corn; eggs; oats; milk and milk products; tomatoes; potatoes; rice; and soy. A professional nutritionist can be consulted for eating a balanced diet. Vitamin C can be helpful in the detoxification process.

HOMEOPATHY

Dr. Samuel Hahnemann, the founder of Homeopathy in 1810, researched and developed remedies based on certain principles. Dr. Hahnemann believed that symptoms are an expression of the body's attempt to heal itself. He stated: "Symptoms are not the disease. Symptoms accompany disease." He sought to treat the underlying problem rather than mask symptoms.

Because of his research Dr. Hahnemann is considered the father of experimental pharmacology. He discovered that when he reduced the dosages of his medicines, they became more powerful. Homeopathic remedies are made up of minute doses of plant, mineral, or animal substances. A minimum dose is 1X, of which the proportion is 1 to 99 and can be extended to 30X, 200X and beyond. His law of infinitesimals states that the smaller the dose, the more effective it will be at stimulating the body's vital forces to heal disease.

Avogadro's Law states that when a medicine is diluted beyond 24X, the medicinal quality is most probably gone. Homeopathy refutes this law.

Hahnemann, as well as homeopathic and alternative physicians of today, talk about a vital force, a power of recovery in the human body. This is a force which reacts to external stimuli. He believed this force creates the symptoms of disease and is vitally important in homeopathic medicine. The homeopathic remedy sets off the chain reaction which the body uses to heal itself.

Hahnemann discovered an interesting phenomenon while doing research on himself. A remedy will cause a certain symptom in a well person. Yet if that remedy is given to a sick person with the same symptom, the sick person will get well.

Homeopathy is practiced extensively in Great Britain. Queen Elizabeth's personal physician is a homeopathic doctor.

HUBBARD METHOD of DETOXIFICATION

The U.S. EPA reports that most Americans have residues of two dozen or more toxic chemicals in their fatty tissues, a major storage site for chemicals which the body cannot metabolize. Regular fasting, cleansing, and other treatment cannot effectively remove these fat-stored substances.

Many pesticides, PCB's and other industrial contaminants, indoor pollutants such as formaldehyde and asbestos, metals such as lead, mercury, and aluminum (from cookware and anti-perspirants), food additives, and many drugs (street drugs, prescribed medications, and anesthetics) are stored in body fat, which is found in most organs and systems of the body including the brain and nervous system. These residues routinely move into the blood, especially during times of physical or mental stress, illness, or extended periods without food. They eventually move back into fat tissue and may remain in the body for months, years, or several decades. The phenomena of spontaneous trips (from LSD) or recurrent illnesses from medicines during times of stress may be caused by this movement of stored chemicals into the circulatory system. Toxic chemicals may also be transferred to the highly sensitive developing fetus or newborn through the placenta or breastmilk.

Persons suffering from chemically-related health problems commonly complain of chronic symptoms, such as headaches, fatigue, inability to concentrate, irritability, rashes, muscular and joint pain, and increased sensitivity to environmental dusts and pollens. As few physicians are trained to recognize chemically-related health problems, and because routine laboratory tests may not detect abnormalities, chemically exposed persons are often told that there is nothing wrong with them, or that their problems are solely of psychological origin. These inaccurate diagnoses are frustrating.

The Hubbard method is a highly sophisticated detoxification program which has been researched and shown to be safe and effective in reducing fat-stored chemicals. It is administered under medical supervision, a necessity when one is rapidly eliminating toxic substances. Some of its main constituents are balanced nutrient support, therapeutic exercise, increased sweat and skin oil excretions in a temperature-controlled, well-ventilated sauna, and therapeutic doses of niacin. The procedure assists the body to move toxic substances out of the fat and eliminate them through the sweat, sebum, urine, and feces.

The regimen is commonly undertaken by persons who have been exposed to chemicals in the work or home environment, including women who wish to reduce chemical levels prior to conception (pregnant women cannot undertake this program), and persons who have completed drug rehabilitation programs but wish to remove stored drug residues from their tissues.

Common benefits reported by persons who have done the Hubbard method of detoxification include remission of chronic symptoms as well as increased energy levels and stamina, improved memory and concentration, softer skin, greater resilience to illness, and an improved sense of well-being.

LIVE CELL THERAPY

Live Cell Therapy is the intramuscular or intradermal injection of suspensions of intact living cells from animal embryonic endocrine glands and other tissues. This therapy stimulates the immune system, improving functioning of vascular, digestive, genital, and respiratory systems. It firms the skin, and returns and preserves vigor, stamina, and vitality. Live cell therapy normalizes hormones, and helps to rejuvenate cells. AIDS patients have sought Live Cell Therapy. Older people seem to feel more vitality in their life from receiving live cell therapy.

Initially Live Cell Therapy may require 48 hours bed rest. After 3 to 4 weeks, the patient will begin to feel stronger. Developed by Dr. P. Niehans in Switzerland, Live Cell Therapy is available in Mexico, contacted through clinics in the United States.

MACROBIOTICS

The main attitude in Macrobiotics is complementing and harmonizing opposites. Food and diet have these opposite qualities, called yin and yang, along with an entire system of life and health. Yin corresponds to expansive foods; yang to contractive foods. In Macrobiotics, the quality of food is not necessarily in its vitamins and minerals, but how yin and yang combine.

The basic principles of Oriental medicine have been used for thousands of years. Macrobiotics was brought to Europe and the USA by Georges Ohsawa, a Japanese man who cured his own tuberculosis using a method relying on traditional Oriental medicine based on yin-yang principles combined with an appreciation of modern nutritional understanding.

Yin foods:

Fruits, drinks, summer foods, sweet, sour or hot foods, purple, blue or green fruits, and vegetables.

Yang foods:

Flesh foods, cereals, some vegetables, foods that are compact and hard, red, yellow, or orange foods, salty or bitter foods, foods which mature in the autumn and winter.

The macrobiotic diet is comprised of whole foods. Most of the food energy comes from complex carbohydrates. Proper cooking methods preserve nutrients and enhance flavor in food.

Macrobiotics stresses that eating must be in harmony with the seasons. That means harmonizing with one's immediate environment by buying food locally in season. Macrobiotic eating develops a natural and instinctive appetite for the right mixture of quality and quantity, avoiding sickness and cravings.

An excess of liquid reduces the efficiency of the kidneys. Therefore, the amount of liquid must be regulated by activity, weather, and individual condition. Processed foods are not used. Food is taken in its most natural form. The emphasis in Macrobiotics is to eat proper amounts. Over-eating is wasteful and demands much of the digestive organs. It is recommended to stop eating before the appetite is satisfied.

Members of the nightshade family are avoided—tomatoes, potatoes, eggplant, green peppers, and tobacco.

Fermented soy products are used regularly—miso, tofu, tamari, and tempeh.

The macrobiotic "way of living" recommends:
- live happily
- be grateful
- retire before midnight and rise early in the morning
- avoid synthetic or wool in contact with skin (clothing and furniture)
- go outdoors often, preferably barefoot; walk on grass and soil
- keep home in good order
- extend love and friendship
- avoid long baths or showers
- scrub whole body with hot damp or dry towel
- avoid chemically perfumed cosmetics
- exercise vigorously
- age, sex, amount of activity, occupation, original constitution, previous

eating patterns, and social environment are all to be considered in new macrobiotic ways.

The emphasis in Macrobiotics is on self-diagnosis and cure.

NATUROPATHY

The Naturopathic principle concerning acute and chronic disease is that when the acute symptoms of childhood are suppressed with drugs and/or superfluous or harmful food, the poisonous waste is driven deeper into the system. The toxins emerge later in a different form. The continued suppression leads to chronic conditions. When undergoing treatment, such as a fast, symptoms long suppressed may rise to the surface and can be eliminated. Naturopathy focuses on the prevention of disease through correct living, eating, and thinking and helps to eliminate toxic conditions from childhood.

Three main principles of naturopathy:

All forms of disease are due to the same cause, namely the accumulation in the system of waste materials and bodily refuse which has been steadily piling up.

The body is always striving for the ultimate good of the individual; self-initiated attempts on the part of the body to throw off the accumulations of waste material may occur and look like illness or disease.

The body contains within itself the power to bring about a return to that condition of normal well-being known as health, provided the right methods are employed to enable it to do so.

Over 150 years ago, as medicine was becoming more structured, some urged a return to simpler, more natural ways of healing and structured those ways. Now called Naturopathy, the approach to healing can involve body-work, acupuncture, acupressure, botanical medicines, nutrition, supplements, counseling, homeo-therapeutics, use of heat, cold, light, water, ultrasound, and electricity. Non-invasive testing, fasting, eliminating drugs, alcohol, tobacco, and coffee, removing toxic waste products, and psycho-emotional reintegration are all part of naturopathic care.

Naturopaths also employ techniques and therapies found in conventional doctors' offices. These include lab tests, physical exams, x-rays, CAT scans, sometimes even minor surgery. The Nature Cure movement of Naturopathy was founded in the 1890s by Dr. John Kellogg, who treated illnesses with natural remedies such as water cures, mineral baths, vegetarianism, fresh air, and sunshine in his Seventh Day Adventist sanitarium in Battle Creek, Michigan. Seventh Day Adventists were at the forefront of nutritional research, vegetarian meat substitutes, breakfast cereals, and natural hospitals.

Dr. Benedict Lust, an MD and an Osteopath, is considered by some as the Father of Naturopathy. He established many health resorts using the above principles of naturopathic healing. Other naturopaths advocated natural programs for health: Gayelord Hauser advised eating live foods. Adolph Just had a back-to-nature program of going barefoot, sleeping outside, and clay compresses. Vincenz Priessnitz and Father Sebastian Kneipp did work in hydrotherapy. Louis Kuhne advocated sun, steam baths, and whole wheat bread. Heinrich Lehmann advocated eliminating salt on foods.

NUTRITION

Nutrition is defined as eating a proper diet, as well as taking supplements—vitamins, minerals, amino acids, enzymes, fatty acids, gland extracts, and digestive aids—while avoiding highly processed or overly-cooked food. The definition of nutrition in this context also includes what you eat, when you eat it, how you prepare it, and how you combine certain foods. Live foods and juices are part of good nutrition, as are aloe vera and spirulina.

Nutrition, or lack of proper nutrition, can affect us in a multitude of ways. Your personality, moods, sex drive, memory, and intellect are all affected by the foods you eat. You are what you eat. Medically accepted knowledge indicates that improper nutrition and diet contribute to vascular disease, gout, diabetes, hypoglycemia, mental illness, constipation, colitis, and increased blood pressure.

Poor eating habits and poor nutrition can lead to poor health and even disease. Dr. Stuart Berger learned through years of research how food can destroy the immune system's proper functioning by eating the wrong food at the wrong time.

Dr. Arthur Kaslow discovered that eating the same foods habitually can cause a stressful malfunction of the immune system. The Kaslow system of eating teaches self-care techniques in eating properly, avoiding foods that the body is sensitive to, and by rotating the diet.

Most holistic health practitioners agree that proper nutrition is a must for prevention of disease and very important in the cure, retardation and/or slowing down of disease already present in the body. Many doctors and osteopaths believe that food can be used as medicine, bringing a person back to health. Fresh vegetables and their juices, as well as fruits and grains, have long-established medicinal properties that can alleviate the symptoms of minor illness.

The foods you eat can make the difference between your day ending with freshness and a delightful evening, or with exhaustion. Scientific studies have found that individual foodstuffs have an effect on sexuality via their chemical constituents. Lack of certain vitamins and minerals may hinder a person's sexual vitality. Food plays an important part of sexual life. When initially eliminating meat from the diet or when beginning food combining, the sex urge may temporarily diminish.

The biochemistry of food and nutrition play an important role in the creation of the diseases anorexia nervosa and bulimia. Once a person is in the vicious cycle of those diseases, the disease can perpetuate itself.

Although many people who are overweight go on endless diets, dieting can encourage weight gain. Fat cells will cause cravings, and will pull more weight towards itself. In other words, the fat cells help to create more fat cells. Dieting itself will not change that. Once off a diet, the body resumes its cravings, addictions, and creating more fat cells.

It may take mega-doses (higher than the recommended daily allowance—usually quite high dosages) of vitamins if a person has been sick or unhealthy for a long time. The immune system may need to be fed large quantities of vitamins in order to heal itself and function properly again. A doctor who is knowledgeable should prescribe mega-vitamins, as improperly diagnosed vitamin therapy is just as dangerous as insufficient nutrition. Because no two people are identical, we are incorrect in assuming that a standard diet will be optimal for all individuals. Each person has his own individual nutritional needs, as well as his own food sensitivities and allergies. One's need for vitamins and minerals is unique. However, Dr. Linus Pauling recommended a minimum of 4 grams (4,000 mg) of Vitamin C per day.

For your health and that of your loved ones, I urge you to watch a 2016 documentary entitled "What's with Wheat?" found on Netflix. Especially if you or they are suffering from auto-immune diseases, digestive upsets, neurological complications like Alzheimer's, autism, depression, and anxiety, or cardiovascular diseases, this is a straightforward discussion of wheat, the ubiquitous wheat industry, GMO wheat, how our bodies cannot utilize gluten, and the many health problems wheat is creating. The information in this video is a massive wake-up call for all of us.

POLARITY

Polarity therapy is the science of stimulating and balancing the life energy in the human body. It is a comprehensive system of health care, including diet, exercise, manipulation, and mental attitude for optimal wellness.

According to Polarity therapy, emotional blockages can be created by childhood conditioning that create chronic negative attitudes. Lack of proper nutrition, dietary imbalance, including choice of foods, quality, quantity, and combinations of foods, how rapidly one eats, and emotional states during eating and digesting can also influence the life energy balance.

The Polarity rebalancing program contains diet, self-help, and stretching exercises while changing one's attitude and personal relationships.

Polarity was developed by Dr. Randolph Stone, (1889-1981), a physician who earned his doctoral degrees in naturopathy, craniopathy, and osteopathy. He also studied western science, natural healing, and the German water cure system. He traveled extensively and studied Eastern healing traditions, then combined Eastern and Western disciplines.

Dr. Stone believed that parts of the body have positive or negative charges and called his healing method Polarity Therapy. Blocked areas create an imbalance in the body's natural energy field, which the polarity practitioner treats. The blockage can be caused by stress, negative thoughts, emotional upset, and lack of proper exercise. The second part of the healing program involves bodywork. The third part of the program is called energy balancing, a non-physical touch.

The purpose of Polarity Therapy is personal transformation by realigning the body to be in harmony with the soul. This somatic therapy enables the patient to look at what he is carrying in his body as a blueprint for his life. The body is a reflection of one's thoughts, beliefs, emotions, and experiences. Polarity Therapy is a chance to release buried treasures and to open up the obstructions, blockages, pain, difficulties, and distortions in the body.

In addition to working with the body, the practitioner supports the patient with verbal communication and reflective listening. One is thus guided into greater awareness, and can re-negotiate what one is holding onto and can therefore let go. Resources for nutrition, exercises, and lifestyle deepen the process of transformation for anyone in any state of health.

PREVENTIVE; INTEGRATIVE; AND HOLISTIC CARDIOLOGY

Heart disease may be preventable. Arterial plaque may be stopped or reversed according to cardiologist Dr. Steve Parcell who reports:

"I spent four years writing a book on the prevention of heart attack and stroke that was published in 2012. The book *Dare to Live* won editor's choice…This is why I am interested in heart disease prevention. I had a heart scan in 2003 that told me I was in the 91st percentile regarding plaque in my coronary arteries (way worse than average). I became very interested in cardiology when I discovered that I was following in my dad's footsteps. My dad had atherosclerosis and hypertension. He died of a heart attack in 1974 at the age of 47. Since 2003 I have been reversing plaque in my patients and preventing heart attack and stroke…The primary cause of heart attacks is atherosclerosis which is a disease of the artery wall. Coronary artery disease is a condition that involves the arteries that supply the heart. When a plaque in an artery becomes too big it can block blood flow to the heart, or, when one of these plaques ruptures, a clot can form which can cause a heart attack or stroke. Coronary artery disease often has no symptoms until your first heart attack. This is why early screening is so important. … patients… are looking for alternatives to prescription drugs, especially statins like Lipitor, Crestor, and Zocor. There are ways to lower blood pressure and cholesterol without drugs." (*Dare to Live*)

Based on research, statin drugs on average only prevent about 30% of heart attacks.

Preventative tests and techniques:
- Cholesterol particle size and number (lipoprotein analysis)
- Advanced cardiovascular risk blood work including genetic markers
- Heart scans to look for calcified plaque
- Carotid artery studies (intimal thickness, ultrasound)
- Echocardiograms to assess heart function
- Endothelial function testing
- Detailed family and medical history
- Physical exam, Exercise plans, Diet plans
- Cholesterol monitoring and blood pressure control

Alternative treatments include:
- EDTA Chelation
- Herbal and nutritional remedies for cholesterol
- IV magnesium
- Naturopathic cardiology

PREVENTIVE AND HOLISTIC DENTISTRY

Preventive dentistry includes proper tooth brushing, flossing, frequent office cleaning, avoiding sugars and processed, refined carbohydrates (sugar, white flour, and white rice) and eating more fresh fruits and vegetables. Prevention of tooth decay, gum disease, and other problems is preferable than suffering the consequences.

The material that causes dental disease, gum bleeding, and cavities, is a whitish-yellow material that sticks to the teeth—called plaque—and is composed primarily of bacteria and food. These bacteria especially love sugar, since it is easily digested by them. As the bacteria that live in the plaque use this food, they give off a waste product that is an acid. It is this caustic acid that can burn a hole in the side of a tooth, and cause decay or a cavity. The acid can also cause the gum tissue to recede and bleed, resulting in gum disease, gingivitis, or pyorrhea.

One concern of preventive dentistry is to make sure that this plaque is removed, before it can do damage, by daily brushing and flossing, correct diet, and periodic visits to the dentist for a more complete cleaning. Ultrasound allows for easier and almost painless teeth cleaning. The plaque almost jumps off the teeth.

According to Dr. Jack Alpan, in The Tune-Up Manual for Humans the correct cause of tooth decay and periodontal disease is an imbalance in calcium to phosphorus ratio in the blood which causes cavities and pyorrhea. The tooth demineralizes into the blood recirculating into the inside of the tooth. He suggests that the individual's ratio be determined and to correct it with diet and supplements.

Dentists perform exams of the mouth, tongue, and jaw for cancer prevention. Saliva tests can also be done to diagnose a wide variety of physical disorders, from cirrhosis of the liver to diabetes and hypertension.

Another concern of a preventive dentist is mercury poisoning from the mercury/silver amalgams (fillings) in your teeth. These fillings give off mercury in the form of gas, ions, and ground-down particles. Dentists can remove these silver amalgams and replace them with composite fillings of porcelain and/or gold.

TMJ, or Temporomandibular Joint Dysfunction, is a problem of the joint linking the upper and lower jaws. This problem, which causes headaches, neck, ear and mouth problems, dizzy spells and pain can be skillfully treated by a holistic dentist.

Hypnosis is being used for pain control, especially for people who are allergic to the various pain-killers (novocaine, zylocaine, etc.). Hypnosis is shown to alter consciousness, change blood pressure, and even decrease salivation and bleeding. It can be used to eliminate thumb sucking and nail biting. Post-hypnotic suggestions can be given to avoid a headache, decrease pain after dental work, and to prepare for the next visit.

Acupuncture can be used for anesthesia. Homeopathic substances can be used to control anxiety, promote healing, prevent infection, control bleeding, and promote the re-growth of dental structure.

Dental implants are available for the denture patient who cannot adjust to dentures or whose gums have receded.

Sonic devices can determine electronically the depth of a periodontal pocket or the length of a root canal.

Fiber optic lights conduct light directly into your mouth for better visibility, can be beamed directly into a nerve canal, and are small enough to enter a tooth socket to locate a tiny broken root tip, Tooth banks are utilized for freezing an extracted tooth for a year or more for implantation later on. Using this technique, it is possible to extract a poorly positioned tooth, along with its root tissue, and reinsert it at a different time.

P.S. While writing this book, I met a man who told me that he and his wife went to a holistic dentist, had all their mercury fillings removed and had them replaced with new composite fillings. He said he noticed afterwards that he felt more alert and energetic than ever before. His wife's health improved dramatically and she no longer suffered from many allergies.

PREVENTIVE AND HOLISTIC MEDICINE

The doctors of today spend nearly one-third of their time treating patients who have chronic, degenerative diseases: arthritis, heart disease, and diabetes. There are no trouble-free means to cure these disorders. Prevention, then, becomes essential.

Because of the Korean War casualties, it was discovered that some diseases are not simply a disease of the elderly. Young American soldiers who were killed were found to be developing coronary heart disease and arteriosclerosis. Doctors found that these diseases take a long time to develop and preventive measures can be taken to avoid or lessen the effects.

Medicine began to penetrate the mysteries of disease and to gain understanding of the interrelationships of mind and body. It explored the influence and mechanisms of heredity in disease. It established the mechanisms of body chemistry and of inborn chemical error. It allied itself with many other sciences from physics and biochemistry, new electronic equipment, and test tube procedures for detecting and monitoring disease. Preventive medicine began to grow and develop with this new knowledge. Understanding the intricacies of the body's chemistry led to new preventive care and to correct a severe problem at the beginning.

Emotional and mental problems were found to affect health. Occupational factors began to be considered. High-risk life styles, such as smoking, obesity, high pulse rate, and low physical activity were seen to play a part in certain diseases.

Racial and social groups have a special propensity to certain illnesses. Calculating risks for various diseases in various groups and people led to monitoring those people regularly. Diabetes is a disease in which the beginning stages can be seen in chemical imbalances. Kidney failure patients were found to have bacteria in their urine which could be detected when they were children, long before the kidneys failed and the patient had to undergo painful dialysis.

What does a preventive physician do?

A thorough and extensive past medical and family history is taken; job, work habits, and living habits, so that health hazards can be corrected.

Any physical complaints will be followed up on, and any mental or emotional problems will be outlined and discussed. Your preventive physician will count on you to explain your symptoms completely, and to consider any harmful habits or behaviors. Since your body is different from other bodies, it will be important for you to be aware of, and report on any problems, you feel.

Tests will be recommended, among them non-invasive tests.

Prevention includes taking responsibility for your own health. Changing your habits and observing the effect of those changes, as well as suggestions for other corrections will be recommended. These habits may include overeating, smoking, improper medication, lack of exercise, imbibing alcohol, using tobacco, and living recklessly—to name a few.

Subtle indications of possible problems will be acted upon, rather than waiting for a disease to become established.

It is the patient himself who will tell the doctor he is sick or thinks he is sick. It will then be up to the preventive physician to determine what the problem is, and treat it accordingly. Any complaints will be considered valid.

Preventive medicine includes techniques to prevent drastic diseases and illnesses, such as mental illness, diabetes, and arthritis, and vascular disease, which results in heart attacks and strokes. Less serious illnesses such as colds, flu, hypoglycemia, and gout can be dealt with as well.

Some of these preventive techniques include, but are not limited to: Chinese Medicine, meditation, yoga, herbs, body manipulation and bodywork. The power of the mind can be harnessed to bring relief, and even possibly, a cure. Rolfing, acupressure, polarity, and chiropractic help to align the body and its energy. Nutrition and orthomolecular medicine can add essential nutrients to the body. These are only a few of the alternative methods that are available today to prevent and relieve illness.

Nutritional awareness is important in prevention: eating proper foods, avoiding highly-processed, overly-refined, and over-cooked foods, proper combining of various foods, and perhaps even food rotation must be considered. Cancer prevention advocates encourage eating foods from the cruciferous family of vegetables, avoiding diets high in bad fats, and eating plenty of high-fiber foods.

Preventive medicine is also for people who are well, to optimize their health physically and psychologically. Boredom, unhappiness, depression, tension, and anxiety can lead to disease by lowering the body's resistance. If a patient is aware of emotional problems, there is a good chance to avoid illness altogether and to remain healthy and happy.

Dr. John Travis runs a Wellness Research Center. His findings are that certain practices are important to preventing disease, illness, and unhappiness:

- Knowing what your real needs are and how to get them met.
- Expressing emotions in ways that communicate clearly what you are experiencing to other people.
- Acting assertively and not passively or aggressively.
- Enjoying your body by means of adequate nutrition, exercise, and physical awareness.
- Being engaged in projects that are meaningful to you and reflect your most important inner values.
- Knowing how to create and cultivate close relationships with others.
- Responding to challenges in life as opportunities to grow in strength and maturity, rather than feeling beset by problems.
- Creating the life you really want, rather than just letting life happen to you.

- Relating to troublesome physical symptoms in ways that bring improvement in condition as well as increased knowledge about yourself.
- Enjoying a basic sense of well-being through times of adversity.
- Knowing your own inner patterns—emotional and physical—and understanding "signals" that your body gives you.
- Trusting that your own personal resources are your greatest strength for living and growing.
- Experiencing yourself as a wonderful person.

Any symptoms need to be diagnosed by a qualified health practitioner. That medical person can recommend changes that are suitable, such as diet, lifestyle, herbs, other remedies, and mental health practices.

Hyperbaric oxygen treatment may be one method used by holistic and preventive physicians. Hyperbaric oxygen therapy (HBOT) is breathing 100% oxygen while under increased atmospheric pressure in a specialized chamber. Certain infections, wounds, carbon monoxide poisoning, and inter-cranial abscesses are a few of the problems treated with HBOT.

PSYCHONEUROIMMUNOLOGY

The immune system must be strengthened not only by proper nutrition and exercise but by properly utilizing the mind. The mind can be used to fight off invaders to the body.

Psychoneuroimmunology is the study of how the mind, the nervous system, and the immune system are interconnected. Kirk Johnson suggests that grief, loneliness, poor self-esteem, and unhappiness can be major contributors to illness. Increasing evidence shows that state of mind can control the state of disease, with the nervous system serving as mediator.

The immune system is responsible for keeping us well, as well as combating disease and sickness. Therefore, many types of disease and illness can benefit from healing attitudes.

Dr. Carl Simonton used this method extensively in his cancer clinics. Using imagery and other mind power techniques to fight different forms of cancer, patients achieved startling success.

The immune system is subject to the mind's whims. Thinking and state of mind can enhance the growth and production of T-cells, which are important in locating and combating invaders to our body in the form of bacteria, fungus, pollens, etc. Positive and happy thoughts can increase production of such chemicals as interferon, interleukin-I, and endorphins, which increase peace of mind, while preventing and combating disease. Negative thinking, on the other hand, can suppress the immune system entirely, leaving the body open to all kinds of problems.

TMJ—TEMPOROMANDIBULAR JOINT DYSFUNCTION THERAPY

The temporomandibular is the joint that attaches the upper and lower jaws. TMJ dysfunction is an improper relationship of the lower jaw to the upper jaw creating symptoms. This problem can be caused by a poor bite, tooth loss and consequent re-shifting, poorly fitting dentures, injury to the jaw, misalignment of the muscles and bones, and tension.

TMJ dysfunction can create head pain, headaches, eye, mouth, ear, jaw, and neck problems, dizzy spells, teeth clenching, soreness, and throat discomfort. This problem can be corrected by an osteopath or chiropractor trained in TMJ therapy. Sometimes a holistic dentist can treat this problem with adjustment and massage. TMJ may require dental work, new dentures, or a splint to correct the bite.

ULTRASOUND THERAPY

Ultrasound is a healing modality as well as a non-invasive diagnostic testing device. Surgeons are able to perform surgery in the parts of the body that used to be inaccessible using high-frequency sound waves. For non-surgical uses, the intensity is lower.

Chiropractors use an ultrasound machine to break up the fluid in muscles, and alleviate muscle stress which is throwing vertebrae out of alignment. Heat is generated as the sound waves rub against cell molecules and cause them to vibrate while it massages the painful tissue. Ultrasound depolymerizes— loosens the glue in long-chained protein molecules—so these tissues become more flexible. Thus, tendons and muscles that are experiencing spasm and are acutely painful, making motion difficult, can become flexible once again.

Other therapeutic uses of ultrasound are for arthritis, tendonitis, and bursitis. Holistic dentists use ultrasound for teeth cleaning and scaling.

WATER THERAPY (HYDROTHERAPY): SPA THERAPY

Water is a natural medicine that helps the whole body. Water therapy, also known as hydrotherapy, consists of using water in many ways and in many forms for healing.

The ancient Romans used hydrotherapy, as did the Babylonians, Egyptians, Turks, and Greeks. Dr. Semmelweis, a Hungarian physician, used various water treatments for disease and illnesses. He was the first doctor to practice washing his hands between seeing patients. Dr. John Kellogg used hydrotherapy in his famous Battle Creek sanitarium.

The therapeutic uses of water are:

- as a restorative and tonic
- for injuries
- to relieve pain
- for minor bums
- to reduce fever
- to induce perspiration
- as a diuretic
- as an antiseptic
- as an elimination
- as a laxative
- as an emetic
- to raise body temperature
- as a stimulant
- as an anesthetic
- as a sedative
- as an antispasmodic
- to relieve thirst
- for buoyancy
- for mechanical effects
- for cleansing internally and externally

The three kinds of water used are liquid, steam, and ice. This therapy can be used in varying temperatures and pressures. Water can be used internally—douche, drinking, enemas, bidet, ear or nose bath. It can be used externally in baths, hot and cold showers, body compresses or packs, hot water bottles, ice packs, or steam.

Other forms of water therapy are fasting, colonics, hot and cold baths, steam baths, saunas, jacuzzis, hip or sitz baths, epsom salt baths, mud packs, mineral baths, wraps in wet sheets, hot and cold foot baths, steam inhalations, hot and cold compresses, sea water therapy, showers, and snow therapy.

Cold compresses to the body cause perspiration and help to eliminate toxic substances, especially when the compress covers the trunk. Water therapy helps aches and pains, relieves respiratory troubles, and aids in indigestion. Hydrotherapy treats arthritis, high blood pressure, and aids in greater resistance to infections. Water can be combined with air baths and sun baths.

SPA THERAPY

A spa is a place where nature has decided to bring forth a spring whose water is either hot or has an unusually high mineral content, preferably both. The chief minerals in spa water are sodium, calcium, magnesium, bicarbonate, and sulfate. These minerals enter the body through the skin and help restore health. The water is also used for drinking, bathing, and underwater exercise.

The healing waters are beneficial for rheumatic complaints, intervertebral disc troubles, and post-traumatic injuries following accidents. The atmosphere is relaxed and comfortable. The environment surrounding a spa contains negative ions, which assist in healing.

Spas have been popular in Europe for centuries and are famous for healing. In the U.S., spas are growing rapidly as health resorts, including other types of water therapy, nutrition, exercise, aroma therapy, body work and other holistic and preventive health methods. People with heart problems or low blood pressure should check with their doctors first before using saunas or Jacuzzis.

P.S. A few of my friends and I went to a hot springs and spa. Two of the women undertook a routine that was greatly rejuvenating and energy enhancing. First, they took a cold shower, then went and sat in the sauna for a while. Then they immersed themselves in a cold tub of water for a few minutes, then back to the hot sauna. This hot/cold procedure was repeated a few times. Afterwards their faces glowed, they reported their energy was higher than ever, and they felt clean inside as well.

Water, water everywhere, but not a drop to drink

Until I researched this category, I had never really given much thought to water therapy, although I drink water frequently as medicine. I was so excited writing about therapeutic uses of water that I immediately took a hot bath using packaged minerals I had bought at a spa.

As I sat soaking, I remembered the poor quality of the drinking and bathing water in my city. Several years ago, I had an extensive water filtration, cleansing, and purifying system installed in my home. Although this system is not as good as naturally pure water, it was better than drinking and washing with the chemicals, sewage, bacteria, and other pollutants that are in my city's water.

In 1988, just before the first edition of this book came out, I was reading extensively about the drought that was sweeping across the United States. For a while we had been complacent on-lookers to Africa and other dry, dusty areas. Now we were in the same deadly struggle for water. While finishing the 2nd edition of this book, the US has been increasingly experiencing drought and lack of rainfall in various regions.

Rain has always symbolized health and growth to me. I love the feeling after a rainfall of being cleansed and refreshed, calmer and more peaceful inside, due to the healing energy of negative ions. Being a gardener, I am extremely conscious of rain water and its effects. Following the disaster at Chernobyl in April 1986, I planted my organic garden. Using the timetable from the Farmer's Almanac, rain generally falls just after planting. Right on schedule the rain came and continued for about a week. Under normal conditions, the seeds germinate quickly and grow lushly with the nourishing spring rain. That fateful spring, though, the rain must have had harmful qualities in it, maybe even radioactivity. My newly sprouting crop died. Other plants and trees also suffered and looked horrible after the rain, as though they were going to perish, too. I was frightened, looking at my destroyed vegetables and distressed garden. Should I plant again, and if I did, would the next rain also be as damaging? For months, I felt sluggish and irritable, as did many people I talked to. Since rain adds negative ions to the atmosphere and creates a calming sensation, why didn't the rain create negative ionization that spring? What had happened to the rain?

Fortunately, my next planting was more successful. The spring of 1988 was productive and rain once again bestowed its tranquil qualities. However, the memory of that ominous rain was shocking.

BODYWORK

Bodywork is any therapeutic technique that involves working with the human body in a form involving energy medicine, manipulative therapy, and/or breath work. The goal of bodywork techniques is to assess or improve posture and remove pain, while promoting awareness and overall health. Bodywork is a perfect therapy by itself as well as a wonderful adjunct to any other therapy, whether traditional or non-traditional. Human beings tend to store injury, hurts, fears, traumas, and other memories in the cells and parts of the body as sensations. Bodywork can assist by bringing to conscious awareness negative feelings and memories, then releasing them from the body.

Bodywork is excellent for working on physical stress and tensions held in the body, as well as for pain, injuries, eliminating toxins through the circulatory and lymphatic system, and to facilitate and speed up the healing process.

Bodywork may initially generate apprehension. To have a stranger touch your body may stimulate negative thoughts and feelings, which is not uncommon, as well as the concern about possible discomfort. However, the positive experiences usually far outweigh any concerns you may have. Many bodyworkers will ask you to remove only the clothing you are comfortable with shedding. Your body is then draped with sheets. Be sure to discuss with your bodyworker any concerns you have regarding nudity, what you are and are not comfortable with, how they will drape your body during the session, and how your body will be exposed. Trager is one form of bodywork in which you remain fully clothed.

Are you worried about pain? Bodywork runs the gamut of touch, from placing hands over the body without touching (in a certain form of Polarity therapy) to very deep tissue manipulation as in Lomi or Rolfing. You always have the option to determine how deeply your bodywork will go into your muscles and tissues. If you want a nurturing touch instead of therapeutic, that's okay, too. If your practitioner doesn't ask what your preferences are, then tell him/her yourself.

If your desire is to avoid deep tissue bodywork altogether, then I would advise you avoid those techniques that specialize in that type of touch. One reason you may wish to avoid deep tissue work is that you are already in a great deal of pain. Sometimes you may require a few sessions to work out the kinks and decrease pain before you can tolerate more intense pressure. Be sure to discuss this with your bodyworker.

Bodywork is be a delicate, highly personal matter. The final authority is you, the person receiving treatment, as to whether or not the type of body-work is appropriate for you, and if the practitioner treats you in a way that is suitable and comfortable.

ACUPRESSURE

Acupressure is a technique similar to acupuncture. The main principle of acupressure is that disease is due to an imbalance in the flow of chi (energy) throughout the body. Acupuncture and acupressure points have been well known in China for about 2,500 years and are believed to correspond to specific organs and areas of the body. These places of correspondence are known as meridians. In treatment, physical pressure is applied to particular meridians in order to clear blockages.

Pressure may be applied by hand, fingers, elbow, or with various devices. Once the point is located, it cannot be mistaken, as it is highly sensitive and the feeling is different from the surrounding tissue.

When doing acupressure, the practitioner generally places the tip of her index or second finger, or thumb on the point. A small object such as a pencil eraser can be used instead of a fingertip. The point will be stimulated from one to five minutes at a time. The pressure that is applied should be as much as the individual can comfortably tolerate.

Relief can last from a few minutes to several hours or days. Acupressure can be obtained from a practitioner or used as a self-help technique for relief of pain. In its Western form, shiatsu has largely taken over acupressure.

Acupressure, although a precise science, is simple to learn. It is easy to merge with other forms of bodywork, like massage therapy and chiropractic.

Some of the problems that are relieved with acupressure are: headaches, including migraines; menstrual cramps; toxic buildup in joints and muscles; pain; TMJ; muscle spasms and digestive problems; reducing nausea, vomiting, and stomach aches; as well as for alleviating lower back pain.

ACUPUNCTURE

Acupuncture is a technique from Chinese medicine that can be traced back at least 2,500 years. The general theory of acupuncture is based on the premise that there are patterns of energy flow (chi) flowing through the body in channels that are essential for health. Disruptions of this flow are believed to be responsible for disease. Chi affects both substance (oxygen, carbon dioxide, and nutrients) as well as functionality (heart, kidneys, liver, and so on). The terminus of the channels on the body's surface are acupuncture points. The flow of chi can be disrupted by imbalances in the body which may result in illness and disease.

Traditional Chinese medicine diagnoses the cause of internal disease (yin/yang imbalance) within the body. The imbalance is remedied by tapping into the chi and balancing it by stimulation of acupuncture points.

Acupuncture is most understood in the West by the insertion of thin, sterilized needles into the skin which stimulate the chi at certain points. The practitioner slowly twirls the needles gently, and leaves them in the skin for 10-30 minutes. Sometimes electrical stimulation is used in conjunction with the needles, by attaching electrodes to them.

Other types of treatment can be done on the acupuncture points. Moxibustion is a form of heat therapy using mugwort on or near the skin.

Another method is called cupping, where a glass or bamboo cup is held over the skin, then heat is applied creating a vacuum. The heat is then allowed to travel directly into the acupuncture points.

To diagnose a problem, the acupuncturist will examine the tongue, listen to the speech and lungs, and feel the pulse. Applied kinesiology (muscle testing) can determine if certain channels are weak or underactive, thus disturbing an organ or function of the body. Chinese herbs may be recommended with, or instead of, acupuncture. Diet and exercise as adjunct therapies are also stressed.

Acupuncture can be employed for all manner of problems or pain and can be used for anesthesia in dentistry and in childbirth as well.

ALEXANDER TECHNIQUE

Alexander technique is a method designed to allow the body to move in a more relaxed and comfortable manner, the way nature intended. People can unconsciously misuse their bodies when standing, sitting, lying down, and during activity. F.M. Alexander developed his technique as an educational process to develop the ability to realign posture and to avoid unnecessary muscular tension.

Alexander believed the individual's self-awareness could be inaccurate, resulting in unnecessary muscular tension such as when standing or sitting with body weight unevenly distributed, holding one's head incorrectly, walking or running inefficiently, and responding to stressful stimuli in an exaggerated way. Alexander said that those who habitually misused their muscles could not trust their innate feelings when carrying out activities or responding to emotional situations.

This technique shows clients how they mistreat themselves and helps them learn new patterns of holding and moving the body. Actions such as sitting, squatting, lunging, or walking are often selected by the teacher to retrain the client. Other actions may be selected for the client, tailored to their interests, work activities, hobbies, computer use, lifting, driving, or performance in acting, sports, speech, or music.

The teacher helps the client to identify and eliminate the harmful habits built up over a lifetime of stress and learn to move more freely. The practitioner touches and guides the client's body, teaching a correct relationship of body parts while the client experiences a new sense of movement. The practitioner uses light touch with moderate to high interaction between her and the client during a session using awareness, releasing inhibition, conscious control, and practice to relearn everyday functions.

The method brings a sense of light and effortless movement. Joint and muscle problems may be alleviated, along with improved breathing, circulation, vision, lowered blood pressure, deeper sleep, and increased cheerfulness. The technique can alleviate repetitive strain injury or carpal tunnel syndrome, a backache or stiff neck and shoulders, or discomfort when sitting at the computer for long periods of time.

The Alexander technique is particularly beneficial for singers, musicians, actors, dancers, golfers, tennis players, or swimmers, especially if they feel they are not performing at full potential.

ASTON-PATTERNING; ASTON KINETICS

Aston-Patterning incorporates the idea that stress or an injury will cause an imbalance. The body adjusts itself to the imbalance, causing more tension, which becomes locked into the body over time.

Judith Aston was a dancer, a certified Rolfer and a movement facilitator with the San Diego Gestalt Institute. She worked with Dr. Ida Rolf who was the director of the Structural Patterning Institute which used patterning in conjunction with structural integration. Ms. Aston felt that Rolfed bodies tended to look alike and that Rolfing was often painful. She believed that better results could be achieved with less effort and pain and so created a new form of bodywork which is now called Aston-Patterning.

This method includes lessons which consist of a step-by-step process of changing one's movement patterns. Each lesson is created according to the individual's needs. Clients become aware of body use in everyday situations like standing, sitting, and walking. As awareness increases, new movement patterns are introduced. The goal is that each client becomes aware of the patterns he or she holds on to mentally, emotionally, and physically. As the body becomes more balanced, the mind also becomes more centered.

Aston-Patterning includes both massage and movement, with feedback from the client. The touch ranges from light to intense.

BIOENERGETICS

Bioenergetics is a therapeutic technique to help a person get in sync with his body and to help him enjoy to the fullest degree possible the life of the body. This emphasis on the body includes sexuality and more basic functions of breathing, moving, feeling, and self-expression. The idea of grounding, making sure a patient has a sense of his feet planted firmly on the ground, being in touch with reality, his body, and his sexuality is one of the cornerstones. Breathing is crucial, as is character analysis.

The benefits of Bioenergetics are inner harmony, feeling free, and opening a person to life and love by discovering the self. In addition, it helps reduce pain and tension in the body, heal headaches, increase sexual health, and eliminate fears.

Bioenergetics has its base in Reichian therapy. However, when Reich began to explore Orgone energy and moved away from physical bodywork and character analysis, Dr. Alexander Lowen broke from Reich and created Bioenergetics.

BIOFEEDBACK and NEURO-FEEDBACK

Biofeedback is a method that uses the mind to control a body function that the body normally regulates automatically, such as skin temperature, muscle tension, heart rate, or blood pressure.

When a client is first learning biofeedback, they will have sensors attached to the body and to a monitoring device. This provides instant feedback on a body function like skin temperature. The biofeedback therapist will then teach the client physical and mental exercises that can help control the function. The results are displayed on the monitor while the client learns how to control that function. The monitor beeps or flashes when the desired change in that body function—such as increasing skin temperature or reducing muscle tension—is achieved.

Biofeedback may be used to improve health, performance, and the physiological changes that often occur in conjunction with thoughts, emotions, and behavior. Eventually, these changes may be maintained without the use of extra equipment, for no equipment is necessarily required to practice biofeedback.

Neurofeedback (EEG) is the voluntary regulation of brain wave activity. It is a learned response, with applications including the modulation of arousal levels, regulating sleep/wake cycles, dealing with cognitive processes, processing sensory information, correcting inappropriate motor responses, controlling moods and emotions and helping deal with memory issues. This method may be helpful for PTSD and complex PTSD and may take up to 30 sessions for total results.

CHIROPRACTIC and NON-FORCE CHIROPRACTIC

Chiropractic is a form of alternative medicine developed by D.D. Palmer and is concerned with the diagnosis and treatment of mechanical disorders of the musculoskeletal system, especially the spine. Proponents believe that such disorders affect general health via the nervous system. The main chiropractic treatment technique involves manual therapy, especially spinal manipulation therapy, and manipulations of other joints and soft tissues. Chiropractic is a health profession focused on treating spinal and musculoskeletal problems primarily through manual manipulation. A chiropractor does not prescribe medication, but relies on a variety of manual therapies, including spinal manipulation, mobilization, as well as adjunctive therapies, to improve function and provide pain relief.

Non-force chiropractic—In 1923 Dr. VanRumpt, while still a student at the National College of Chiropractic, became interested in a different approach to structural analysis and correction. He initially found that the mere pressure of spinal palpation on his patients often resulted in unexpected structural, symptomatic, and physiologic changes. He soon felt that a low force was not only an alternative to the more forceful chiropractic methods but might even surpass them in power and results. Non-force adjustments are comprehensive and includes spine, pelvis, cranial, shoulder, upper and lower extremities, TMJ, and organ reflexes. Non-force may be safely applied to babies, geriatrics, post-surgical patients, and those who have disc herniations.

Although it took many years to be accepted by the insurance industry, chiropractic and non-force chiropractic are generally covered by insurance, Medicare and Medicaid.

CRANIAL ADJUSTMENT

The skull serves two purposes. One is to protect the brain. The cranial bones are also responsible for normal nerve and energy patterns through the body. The cranial bones are designed to accommodate very slight movement. Dr. W. Sutherland, an osteopath, originally detected this motion and devised the cranial adjustment therapy. When the practitioner is adjusting the bones, the patient may feel that the osteopath's hands are moving very slowly or are undulating. Correction is made by pressing on the cranial bone in a very specific pressure and direction while the patient breathes in a pattern that assists the correction. The patient becomes aware of a distinct reduction of tension physically and perhaps even emotionally. Cranial therapy can be used on infants, as it is very gentle. Sometimes patients fall asleep during treatment.

Trauma and injuries are not limited to the spine and extremities. The skull is comprised of 13 bones that are joined together with sutures. Although the sutures cannot be pulled apart, the bones in the skull can be knocked out of their proper alignment. The onset of health problems may be the result during childbirth including birth trauma and forceps birthing; along with falls in infancy; the incidence of head injuries due to baseball bats, swings, balls, pucks, fists, sports injuries, and auto and industrial accidents. In fact, microscopic research has demonstrated that nerves from the skull and spine control the immune system down to the cellular level.

Unfortunately, most patients do not receive adequate care for skull and spine injuries. Their conditions deteriorate and result in chronic debilitating health problems. When the cranial bones are misaligned, this is known as subluxation. If cranial subluxations that resulted from a head injury are not corrected, symptoms will persist and become chronic, causing a lifetime of pain, an endless emotional roller coaster, cognitive disorders, and cognitive difficulties resulting in a substandard level of life and health.

Cranial therapy can be applied to problems with migraine headaches, vertigo, whiplash injuries to the neck, as well spinal and limb pain.

DEEP TISSUE WORK

Deep tissue refers to a type of pressure and depth of massage or manipulation used in bodywork. Tissue refers to the muscles, ligaments, and connective tissue in the body. The pressure to the body can range from firm to intense, and may sometimes be painful.

Deep tissue work is a type of massage therapy which uses firm pressure and slow strokes to reach deeper layers of muscle and fascia, the connective tissue surrounding muscles. This method is used for chronic aches and pain and contracted areas such as a stiff neck and upper back, low back pain, leg muscle tightness, and sore shoulders.

While some of the strokes may feel the same as those used in Swedish massage therapy, deep tissue massage isn't the same as having a regular massage with deep pressure. At the beginning of the massage, lighter pressure is generally applied to warm up and prep the muscles. Specific techniques are then applied.

The most common techniques include:
- Stripping—deep, gliding pressure along the length of the muscle fibers using the elbow, forearm, knuckles, and thumbs
- Friction—pressure applied across the grain of a muscle to release adhesions and realign tissue fibers

Deep tissue work is used to break up scar tissue and physically break down muscle knots or adhesions—bands of painful, rigid tissue that can disrupt circulation and cause pain, limited range of motion, and inflammation. Deep tissue work is done in order to remove deep-seated problems, toxins, and even to restructure the body. Some of the different forms of bodywork which may utilize deep tissue work are Rolfing, Lomi, Shiatsu, and Aston-Patterning.

EGOSCUE METHOD

The Egoscue Method, developed by Pete Egoscue, has offered non-medical pain relief since 1971. This easy and gentle method has a high success rate without the use of drugs, surgery, or manipulation. The patient is taught how to regain control of his health without becoming dependent on another person or a machine.

The metabolism and immune system as well as every other system in the body are directly linked to posture. The Egoscue Method is basically a set of prescribed stretches utilizing gravity that puts one's body back into a natural alignment and function of posture. Rather than using manipulation, massage, or any other technique, Egoscue strengthens the appropriate muscles which then can be used to pull the body back into alignment.

The body has an amazing ability to heal itself. The body is made to move and, according to Egoscue, there are zero design flaws. The Egoscue method's approach is to eliminate pain while striving to return the patient to as close as possible to that flawless design. Egoscue helps athletes return to competition pain free while decreasing their chances of future injury, by using the Egoscue Method to enhance performance and extend their careers.

For someone who wants to increase energy level and improve overall health, Egoscue helps patients to tap into the body's ability to not only rid itself of pain, but also heal itself of disease and sickness.

FELDENKRAIS

Some people come to the Feldenkrais method as a form of self-exploration, to learn more about themselves and enhance their general well-being. Others arrive to find better ways of dealing with specific problems such as stroke, spinal injuries, back problems, or other forms of chronic pain, physical and emotional distress. The method doesn't treat these conditions in any medical sense, but helps the patient find new ways of responding to the condition, leading to greater ease and comfort than was previously experienced.

The Feldenkrais method considers problems and illness as faulty body education rather than being sick. Habitual brain responses hamper movement and therefore creativity and energy is limited. Using Feldenkrais, the movements of the body are re-educated and responses that are habitual are eliminated.

Dr. Moshe Feldenkrais was an engineer and applied physicist, who had a knee injury from playing soccer. He was given a 50/50 chance of regaining his health through surgery. He decided he would learn how to walk all over again. He studied physiology, anthropology, anatomy, and psychology and continued to master martial arts and yoga, in order to restore his normal functioning. Based on his research he developed this unique body-centered learning process with gentle movement sequences which emulate the exploratory learning that is natural to infants.

One form of the method is bodywork with individual lessons and therapy called Functional Integration, performed by a trained Feldenkrais practitioner. The other are movement lessons done in a class called Awareness through Movement.

FRANKLIN METHOD

Eric N. Franklin is a Swiss dancer, movement educator, university lecturer, writer and founder of the Franklin Method, a method that combines creative visualization, embodied anatomy, physical and mental exercises and educational skills. The Franklin method is considered ergonomic training which works on the fascia coupled with dynamic neuro-cognitive imagery.

HELLERWORK

Joseph Heller was an aerospace engineer and a certified Rolfer. Hellerwork is an outgrowth of Rolfing with emphasis on body awareness and movement education as well as deep tissue work. Hellerwork lasts eleven sessions instead of the ten in Rolfing. These sessions are designed to progressively integrate muscle and connective tissue, resulting in optimal health and well-being. The touch is moderate to intense. There is medium to high verbal interaction between the Heller practitioner and the patient. Clients often feel a profound release of both physical and emotional tension.

Benefits include reduced tension and stress, increased flexibility, increased energy, grace and agility, greater sensuality, increased body awareness, and overall improved personal appearance. Hellerwork also helps alleviate sports injuries, curvature of the spine, back pain, headaches, poor posture, and tight neck and shoulders.

LOMI (LOMILOMI)

In the Hawaiian language, the word used traditionally, called lomi, meant "to knead, to rub, or soothe; to work in and out, as the paws of a contented cat." Lomilomi practices varied by family, traditional region, and island. Lomilomi means massage therapist or Hawaiian massage.

The Lomi school was founded in 1970 by Alyssa Hall, MA, Robert Hall, MD, Catherine Heckler MA, Richard Heckler, Ph.D, along with Vincent and Zelita Regalbuto.

Lomi nowadays refers to a form of bodywork which incorporates other approaches to transformation and healing, such as polarity therapy, structural integration, reflexology, gestalt and Reichian therapies, breathing exercises, principles of aikido, as well as yoga and meditation. Lomi blends Eastern disciplines with modern psychological methods. The goal is achieving balance obtained by working with the physical, mental, emotional, and spiritual planes as a whole.

Chronic and acute ailments can be minimized through Lomi—headaches, indigestion, constipation, back pain, and fatigue. The person learns through feedback to become more aware of his feelings and his body. Lomi bodywork is done with a client as opposed to on a client. Client participation is emphasized. Changes occur through the session and, because the client is an active participant, he can constantly confront these changes.

MASSAGE

Massage therapy is probably the oldest method for alleviating pain and the symptoms of disease and for promoting good health. It has a long history in cultures around the world and dates back thousands of years. References to massage appear in writings from ancient China, Japan, India, Arabic nations, Egypt, Greece, and Rome. Hippocrates defined medicine as the art of rubbing.

Massage became widely used in Europe during the Renaissance. In the 1850s, two American physicians who had studied in Sweden introduced Swedish massage therapy in the United States, where it became popular and was promoted for a variety of health purposes. With scientific and technological advances in medical treatment during the 1930s and 1940s, massage fell out of favor in the United States. Interest in massage revived in the 1970s, initially among athletes and dancers.

According to the 2007 National Health Interview Survey, which included a comprehensive survey of use by Americans, an estimated 18 million U.S. adults and 700,000 children had received massage therapy in the previous year. People use massage for a variety of health-related purposes, including pain relief, rehabilitation of sports injuries, stress reduction, increased relaxation, to address anxiety and depression, and aid in general wellness.

Massage is concerned with the laying on of hands and therapeutic touch of the soft tissues. There are three main types of touch in massage:

- Stroking—also known as effleurage; long stroking movements, a gliding movement with a light pressure known to have a relaxing, sedating effect.
- Compression—also known as petrissage; kneading and friction, improves circulation, removal of waste products, breaks up adhesions, dilates blood vessels, improves blood and lymph circulation
- Percussion—cupping, slapping or tapping, vibration or shaking, which affects deeper organs, muscles, arteries, lungs, adrenals, and kidneys and reduces pain.

Legitimate massage had a revival through alternative health care. Many RN's and LVN's have taken massage courses while alternative health care centers in doctor's offices, health spas, and physical therapists often offer therapeutic massage for their patients. Massage therapists are often required to complete 100 or more hours of training and have a membership in a professional massage organization or association in order to be licensed.

ORTHO-BIONOMY

Ortho-bionomy is an innovative system of bodywork which can help discover the self-healing secrets within the body. As a technique, it is capable of initiating deep, spontaneous changes in muscles and joints and releasing tension in a way that doesn't involve experiencing more pain, while improving posture, coordination, and flexibility. A patient can learn how to apply the principles for self-healing. There is a natural easy way to release tension and pain built right into the design of the body.

Ortho-bionomy integrates the body, mind and spirit, initiating personal healing reflexes. It is an effective method of dealing with acute and chronic pain, emotional release, and structural alignment without the use of force or manipulation.

Ortho-bionomy is a gentle method which uses non-forceful movements and comfortable positions to unlock tension and relieve pain. Clients learn how to self-correct their muscular/skeletal problems and pain symptoms. The correction is to adjust the body in the direction of the imbalance rather than forcing the body out of imbalance by opposite movement. Muscles and ligaments are then relaxed and balanced.

With ortho-bionomy the patient gains increased awareness of his body and how to use the body to prevent muscle tension. With that awareness a patient can do exercises on his own to improve the quality of his life.

POLARITY

Polarity therapy is the science of stimulating and balancing the life energy in the human body. It is a comprehensive system of health care, including diet, exercise, manipulation, and mental attitude for optimal wellness.

According to Polarity therapy, emotional blockages can be created by childhood conditioning that creates chronic negative attitudes. Lack of proper nutrition, dietary imbalance, including choice of foods, quality, quantity, and combinations of foods, how rapidly one eats, and emotional states during eating and digesting can also influence the life energy balance.

The Polarity rebalancing program contains diet, self-help, and stretching exercises while changing one's attitude and personal relationships.

Polarity was developed by Dr. Randolph Stone, (1889-1981), a physician who earned his doctoral degrees in naturopathy, craniopathy, and osteopathy. He also studied western science, natural healing, and the German water cure system. He traveled extensively and studied Eastern healing traditions, then combined Eastern and Western disciplines.

Dr. Stone believed that parts of the body possess positive or negative charges, and called his healing method Polarity Therapy. Blocked areas create an imbalance in the body's natural energy field, which the polarity practitioner treats. The blockage can be caused by stress, negative thoughts, emotional upset, and lack of proper exercise. The second part of the healing program involves two kinds of bodywork. The third part of the program is called energy balancing, and is a non-physical touch.

The purpose of Polarity Therapy is personal transformation by re-aligning the body to be in harmony with the soul. This somatic therapy enables the patient to look at what he is carrying in his body as a blueprint for his life. The body is a reflection of one's thoughts, beliefs, emotions, and experiences. Polarity Therapy is a chance to release buried treasures and to open up the obstructions, blockages, pain, difficulties, and distortions in the body.

In addition to working with the body, the Practitioner supports the patient with verbal communication and reflective listening. One is thus guided into greater awareness, and can re-negotiate what one is holding onto and can therefore let go. Resources for nutrition, exercises, and lifestyle deepen the process of transformation for everyone in any state of health.

REFLEXOLOGY

Reflexology is a method which deals with the theory that there are points (reflexes) in the feet and hands which correspond through energy channels to all of the glands, organs, and parts of the body. Reflexology, also known as zone therapy, involves application of pressure to the feet and hands with specific thumb, finger, and hand techniques without the use of oil or lotion.

By applying pressure to reflex areas, a reflexologist is said to remove energy blockages and promote health in the related body area. According to reflexologists, pressure on the reflex points also helps to balance the nervous system and stimulates the release of endorphins that help to reduce pain and stress.

Here are some examples of reflex areas of the foot and corresponding body parts:
- the head is located on the tips of the toes
- the heart and chest are around the ball of the foot
- the liver, pancreas and kidney are in the arch of the foot
- low back and intestines are positioned towards the heel

Although the roots of reflexology go back to ancient Egypt and China, William H. Fitzgerald, an ear, nose, and throat doctor, introduced this concept of zone therapy in 1915. Dr. Fitzgerald brought his discovery of the Chinese method of Zone Therapy to the attention of the medical world. He pointed out that pressure and stimulation of certain zones has a definite effect on bringing about normal physiological functioning in all parts of the zone treated, no matter how remote this area may be from the part upon which the stimulation is exerted. American physiotherapist Eunice Ingram further developed the zone theory in the 1930s into what is known as modern reflexology with seminars offered through the USA, Canada, and other parts of the world.

REICHIAN THERAPY

Reichian therapy is a deep emotional release therapy. Reichian therapy can refer to several schools of thought and therapeutic techniques which originate in the work of psychoanalyst Wilhelm Reich (1897–1957), an Austrian psychoanalyst. Reich spent six years as clinical assistant to Dr. Sigmund Freud, then broke ties with Freud, due to his expounding controversial theories and research.

Reich's therapy is based upon character analysis. The patient becomes more aware of his character in a feeling or experiential way, rather than intellectually. The Reichian therapist points out incongruities in the patient's behavior, then encourages the patient to openly express the repressed positive and negative emotions.

Repressed emotions can become frozen in the body, this is known as armoring. Reichian bodywork deals with the feeling and body reactions that are locked into the body together. The patient is encouraged to make faces, scream, breathe deeply, kick, and throw tantrums in order to release the repressed emotions that have hardened in the body. This then releasing the armoring from the body.

Reichian therapy consists of touching, pressing, and muscular manipulation. Deep massage, working with the patient's facial expressions, pushing down on the patient's chest, and shaking is all done by the therapist. Reichian Therapy is the classical foundation of Somatic Psychology.

Some examples are:

- **Bioenergetic analysis**—combines psychological analysis, active work with the body and relational therapeutic work.
- **Body psychotherapy**—addresses the body and the mind as a whole with emphasis on the relationships between them.

- **Bodywork**—neo-Reichian practitioners attempt to locate and dissolve physically repressed emotions known as body armoring or holding patterns.
- **Vegetherapy**—a type of psychotherapy that addresses the physical manifestations of emotions such as pain, illness, and disease.
  (also see Reichian therapy in PSYCHOLOGY)

ROLFING

Rolfing is a form of bodywork which frees and softens the connective tissue which has become frozen, to support posture, so that as the tissue is freed, the head and neck begin to fall back and ride more directly upon the spine without effort. Rolfing is based on two theories: the human body is an energy mass organized in space and subject to the laws and forces of gravity; and the body is a plastic medium capable of change.

Rolfing aligns this connective tissue, the myofascial structure, which holds the body together. This structure can be changed by adding energy. One method used to change structure is by applying pressure to the tissue.

Rolfing is a process of organizing and balancing the body left to right, front to back, top to bottom, and inside out around a vertical line in the field of gravity, so that one is supported and uplifted by gravitational force rather than torn down by it.

Rolfing is a form of bodywork originally developed by Dr. Ida Rolf (1896–1979) called Structural Integration, and typically delivered as a series of ten hands-on physical manipulation sessions sometimes called the Recipe. Dr. Rolf was also a biochemist at the Rockefeller Institute and was instrumental in developing lecithin. The Recipe is based on Rolf's ideas about how the human body's energy field can benefit when aligned with the Earth's gravitation field. Practitioners combine superficial and deep manual therapy with movement prompts.

Rolfing is based on Rolf's proposition that a human is basically an energy field operating in the greater energy of the earth. Rolf described the body as organized around an axis perpendicular to the earth, parallel to the pull of gravity, and believed the function of the body was optimal when it was organized in that way. She saw the body as continually in a struggle with gravity;

in her view, gravity tends to shorten fascia, leading to disorder of the body's arrangement around its axis and creating imbalance, inefficiency in movement, and pain. Rolfers aim to lengthen the fascia in order to restore the body's arrangement around its axis and facilitate improved movement.

Rolfers integrate the body so that it acts more efficiently as a unit, especially in relationship to gravity and physical laws. The head, thorax, shoulders, pelvis, and legs are aligned vertically to give the patient more balance, while the body is lengthened and straightened. Bones are allowed to readjust themselves to their proper place and their proper relationship to each other. The autonomic system is aligned with the structural system allowing the autonomic system to better function. After Rolfing, the structure is changed, which affects health and well-being. Chronic holding of muscles which demanded energy from the body is released. The patient feels less tired and depressed after Rolfing.

Rolf claimed to have found an association between emotions and the soft tissue. Although Rolfing is not primarily a psychotherapeutic approach to the problems of humans, it does constitute an approach to the personality through the myofascial collagen components of the physical body. Emotional pain can be released, as well as grief, tenseness, and memories.

Some osteopaths were influenced by Rolf, and several of her students became teachers of new forms of bodywork.

SHIATSU

Shiatsu is a form of Japanese bodywork based on traditional Chinese medicine. In the Japanese language, shiatsu means finger pressure. Classical Oriental Medicine views both internal and external influences as the primary cause of illness. To treat a symptom is partial treatment. One must treat the person in entirety while the Shiatsu technique assists the body in healing itself. There are a number of points on the surface of the body where pressure applications produce remarkable results. These points are located at important places over muscles, bones, nerves, blood vessels, and glands of the endocrine system.

The Japanese Ministry of Health defines shiatsu as a form of manipulation by thumbs, fingers, and palms without the use of instruments, mechanical or otherwise, to apply pressure to the human skin to correct internal malfunctions, promote and maintain health, and treat specific diseases. The techniques used in shiatsu include stretching, holding, and most commonly, leaning body weight into various points along key channels, or meridians. Shiatsu techniques include massage using fingers, thumbs, feet and palms, and sometimes elbows, assisted stretching, and joint manipulation and mobilization. To examine a patient, a shiatsu practitioner uses palpation and pulse diagnosis.

Shiatsu is the oldest form of physical therapy and derives from a Japanese massage modality called anma which was adapted from tui na. Tui na is a Chinese bodywork system that arrived in Japan by around 710–793 CE., created in Japan by Buddhist monks. Tokujiro Namikoshi (1905–2000) founded a shiatsu college in the 1940s, and is often credited with inventing modern shiatsu.

TOUCH FOR HEALTH

Touch for Health is a system of balancing posture, attitude, and life energy for greater comfort, vitality, and enjoyment of your life. Touch for Health falls under the branch of alternative therapy known as kinesiology—systems of healing that use manual muscle bio-feedback to determine which stimuli stress the body and how that stress can be decreased. Touch for Health evolved from Chinese Medicine and is a simple and methodical series of techniques whose principle is that the relative strengths of isolated muscles indicate specific organ imbalances. All muscles used in Touch for Health relate to one of the 14 major acupuncture meridians, or energy pathways, while each muscle relates to an organ, gland, function, or body part such as the eyes or ears.

The Touch for Health model does not treat or diagnose symptoms, but works with the energy, lifestyle, and aspirations of the client, offering a safe and effective way to maintain health, enhance well-being, and upgrade performance.

The goal is to balance the body's energy to allow the life force to flow uninterrupted, so that the organism can heal itself and experience optimal health and well-being.

Touch for Health is a synthesis of ancient knowledge of the Chinese acupuncture meridians along with techniques derived from chiropractic, naturopathy, osteopathy, and even person-centered counseling, including acupressure, a variety of touch reflexes, meridian tracing, nutrition, and a variety of mind-body techniques for balancing the subtle energies while focusing on meaningful, personal goals.

Touch for Health is a specific bodywork technique. However, human touch, whether by a professional health care professional or socially, is healing and essential to emotional health, physical well-being, perhaps even life itself. This is why we must caress, we must rock babies, even massage their bodies. Deprived of touch, babies would rather die, and they often do. This lack of touching can also lead to complex PTSD wherein a child feels abandoned and alone, which disrupts proper brain functioning as well as disturbs the central nervous system.

TRAGER

The Trager Approach is an innovative approach to movement education, created and developed over a period of 65 years by Milton Trager, M.D. There are two aspects of the Trager Approach—one in which the client is passive and the other in which she is active. The passive aspect is usually referred to as the tablework, and the active aspect is called Mentastics.

Utilizing gentle, non-intrusive, natural movements, the Trager Approach helps release deep-seated physical and mental patterns and facilitates deep relaxation, increased physical mobility, and mental clarity. These patterns may have developed in response to accidents, illnesses, or any kind of physical or emotional trauma, including the stress of everyday life. A session usually lasts from 60 to 90 minutes. No oils or lotions are used and the client is dressed for comfort, with a minimum of swimwear or briefs, and draped appropriately with sheets.

During the table work session the client is passive and lying on a comfortably padded table. The practitioner moves the client in ways she naturally moves, and with a quality of touch and movement such that the recipient experiences the feeling of moving effortlessly and freely on her own. The movements are never forced so that there is no induced pain or discomfort to the client. Through Trager bodywork the patient learns to recognize and let go of their unconscious physical and emotional holding patterns; to reduce stress, friction, and chronic tension; to increase resiliency, flexibility, and mobility by dissolving old limiting patterns of movement and perceptions of self; to support an expanded capacity for desired self-expression; and to enhance conscious awareness of integration of body, mind, and spirit.

This quality of effortless movement is maintained and reinforced by Mentastics. These are simple, active, self-induced movements which the client can do on her own, during her daily activities. The movements have the same intent as the table work in terms of releasing deep-seated patterns.

For many people, Mentastics becomes a part of their life in taking care of themselves, and relieving themselves of stress and tension. Because many of the effects of the Trager Approach are cumulative, clients most often appreciate and will benefit most from a series of sessions. One of the truly potent aspects of the Trager Approach is the ability to recall the feeling of deep relaxation, and how it feels to move freely and easily.

NON-TOUCH BODYWORK METHODS

CONSCIOUS BREATHWORK (REBIRTHING); PRANAYAMA YOGA

Conscious Breathwork consists of rhythmic breathing or breathing techniques with or without a coach which can remove anxiety, provide deep and lasting healing of emotional pain, release suppressed or blocked emotions, promote profound physical, emotional and mental relaxation, release toxins in the body on a cellular level, increase feelings of connection with others and the universe along with enhanced spiritual awareness, and allow access to unconscious and transpersonal information, clues that provide information to one's life/soul purpose, and the experience of bliss.

QIGONG

Qigong is an ancient Chinese health care system that integrates physical postures, breathing techniques, and focused intention. The word Qigong is made up of two Chinese words. Qi is pronounced chee and is usually translated to mean the life force or vital-energy that flows through all things in the universe. The second word, Gong, pronounced gung, means accomplishment, or skill that is cultivated through steady practice. Together, Qigong means cultivating energy. It is a system practiced for health maintenance, healing, and increasing vitality.

Qigong is an integration of physical postures, breathing techniques, and focused intentions. Qigong practices can be classified as martial arts, medical, or spiritual. All styles have three things in common: they all involve a posture, (whether moving or stationary), breathing techniques, and mental focus. Some practices increase the Qi; others circulate it, use it to cleanse and heal the body, store it, or emit Qi to help heal others. Practices vary from the soft internal styles such as T'ai Chi; to the external, vigorous styles such as Kung Fu. However, the slow gentle movements of most Qigong forms can be easily adapted, even for the physically challenged, and can be practiced by all age groups.

Qigong creates an awareness of and influences dimensions of our being that are not part of traditional exercise programs. Most other forms of exercise do not involve the meridian system used in acupuncture nor do they emphasize the importance of adding mindful intent and breathing techniques to physical movements. When these dimensions are added, the benefits of exercise increase exponentially. The gentle, rhythmic movements of Qigong reduce stress, build stamina, increase vitality, and enhance the immune system. It has also been found to improve cardiovascular, respiratory, circulatory, lymphatic, and digestive functions.

PSYCHOLOGICAL THERAPIES

Which came first? The chicken or the egg? Do we first have negative thoughts, feelings and experiences which later manifest as illness, discomfort, and disease? Or do we have physical problems originating in the body through germs, bacteria, and genetic disturbances which later begin to affect the way we think and behave? Immunologists concur in part with the idea that thought is creative. Positive thoughts can influence our immune system and help it to work properly, secreting substances needed to combat and prevent illness as well as to bring relaxation to the body. These same researchers have found that negative thoughts and attitudes negatively affect the immune system, suppressing those same substances and blocking the proper functioning of our immune system, which can later lead to disease and poor health.

Nature vs. nurture? What seems to be true is that the body and mind are connected and work together, either in harmony or disharmony. Thus one can decide to get psychological assistance to help in the healing of the body through the mind and emotions.

When choosing a counselor or psychotherapist, it can be useful to understand the different therapies used. Although all can be effective, you may find one approach more appealing than another, or find that some approaches are better for a certain area of counseling or psychotherapy than others.

Psychological therapies generally fall into the following categories:
- Behavioral therapies, which focus on cognitions and behaviors
- Psychoanalytical and psychodynamic therapies, which focus on the unconscious relationship patterns that evolved from childhood

- Humanistic therapies, which focus on self-development in present time
- Art therapies, which use creative arts within the therapeutic process
- Family and couples counseling, which look to resolves issues experienced by families and couples

Counseling or psychotherapy often overlaps some of those techniques. Some counselors or psychotherapists practice a form of integrative therapy, which means they draw on and blend specific types of techniques. Other practitioners work in an eclectic way, which means they take elements of several different models and combine them when working with clients.

A counselor must have a degree, be licensed to practice, and have interned a specific number of hours. Degrees can be one of the following: Ph.D. (doctor of philosophy), Psy.D. (doctor of psychology), M.D. (doctor of medicine), LISW (licensed independent social worker), LCSW (licensed clinical social worker), CNS (clinical nurse specialist), LPCC (licensed professional clinical counselor), or MSW (masters in social work).

The methods below are specific tools to support the clinical healing relationship. But there is no replacement for a mature, nurturing therapeutic presence and the ability to engage another suffering human in a safe and trusting relationship where the person feels heard, accepted, and understood.

AFFIRMATIONS

Developing a positive mindset is one of the most powerful life strategies there is. Using positive thinking techniques, visualizations, and positive affirmations, it is possible to achieve whatever you want. Professionals and business people can use these techniques to develop personal power or gain a competitive edge. At a personal level affirmations can transform your life, your health, and renew your joy and passion for life. Imagine waking up each morning, bursting with excitement, energy, and joy for the new day.

Our beliefs define our reality. What we believe about ourselves and life become true for us. Affirmations reprogram one's thinking, and help us to let go of the negative patterns that have been sabotaging us and adopt potent success techniques to bring about what we want.

Are you suffering poor health or facing a healing crisis? Health problems often have a psychological and emotional basis and it is important to investigate any potential causes. By examining and dealing with underlying psychological and emotional issues you can dramatically improve your heath and healing outcomes.

If we expect and believe that life is a struggle for us and that people treat us badly then that is probably what our experience will be. Likewise we can love ourselves and believe that we deserve all good in our lives and have a right to loving healthy relationships. To make changes in our lives we can clear out old negative thoughts of not being good enough or deserving, and nourish ourselves with new constructive and loving thoughts.

People we attract are a mirror of our own inner beliefs about ourselves and the world. You can take charge of your romantic life, supercharge your existing relationship, or attract your perfect new partner. You can learn to accept what you deserve and want in your relationships.

Positive affirmations and positive thinking techniques can help develop a constructive attitude to life, which is an essential element in life success and good health. With this power you can turn failure into success and take success and drive it to a whole new level. Your positive attitude is the fuel for your success.

Sound psychological techniques, your own personal power, and your connection to the universe can create an awesome combination to manifest any change into your life. Affirmations can create new pathways called engrams in the brain which become more powerful than negative programming.

Our Thoughts are Creative. What we think creates our reality.

The universe is infinitely abundant, so you can place your cosmic order with the universe and manifest what you want.

The world is infinitely abundant and your well-being is there for the taking.

One type of affirmation exercise I've practiced for years and which has brought amazing benefits to my life is called "Writing a God Letter." You can find instructions and this essay in my book Cosmic Grandma Wisdom.

ATTITUDINAL HEALING

Principles of attitudinal healing:

- The essence of our being is love.
- Health is inner peace. Healing is letting go of fear.
- Giving and receiving are the same.
- We can let go of the past and the future.
- Now is the only time there is and each instant is for giving.
- We can learn to love ourselves and others by forgiving rather than judging.
- We can become love finders rather than fault finders.
- We can choose and direct ourselves to be peaceful inside regardless of what is happening outside.
- We are students and teachers to each other.
- We can focus on the whole of life rather than the fragments.
- Since love is eternal death need not be viewed as fearful.
- We can always perceive ourselves and others as either extending love or giving a call for help.

Some influential resources:

- *Love is Letting Go of Fear* by Dr. Gerald Jampolsky, Center for Attitudinal Healing
- *Power vs. Force* by Dr. David R. Hawkins
- *The Law of Attraction*, the Abraham-Hicks teachings
- *Things Are Going Great In My Absence* by Lola Jones

BIOENERGETICS

Bioenergetic Analysis (bioenergetics) is a unique and effective psychotherapy system that helps resolve emotional issues by engaging the wisdom of the body in a safe and caring relationship with a trained therapist. Bioenergetics has a long and established history, yet finds itself on the cutting edge of contemporary psychology as rapid advances in neurobiology highlight the intricate and intimate relationship between body and mind. Bioenergetics recognizes that our experiences leave physical imprints from our earliest days of childhood. Our physiological responses to events in our lives are stored in our cells and muscles as well as our minds. Negative stored memories can manifest in a range of problems in adult life, from patterns of failed relationships to illness and chronic pain.

Bioenergetics also recognizes that difficult childhood experiences occur in the context of close relationship with parents and caretakers, and that healing from them requires a nurturing and safe relationship in the present. Bioenergetics invites the release of unconscious holding patterns in the body through breathing, movement, and emotional expression while being supported and protected by a trained and caring therapist. People who have experienced this combination of safe relationship and full expression of themselves through their bodies testify that they have renewed energy they can apply toward healthy pleasure and purpose in life.

BIO-FEEDBACK; NEUROFEEDBACK

Every animal is a self-regulating system owing its existence, it stability, and most of its behavior to feedback controls from the brain, the heart, the circulatory system, and the different muscle groups. Bio-feedback is the process of gaining greater awareness of physiological functions initially using instruments that provide information on the activity of those same systems, with a goal of being able to manipulate them at will. Some of the processes that can be controlled include brainwaves, muscle tone, skin conductance, heart rate, and pain perception.

A bio-feedback machine is a monitoring device that is used to extend the five senses, creating, in effect, a new sense that allows awareness of mind/body processes that were previously inaccessible to the conscious mind. The instruments amplify and interpret the feedback into signals that the patient can recognize, such as a flashing light, a steady tone, squiggle of a pen, or the movement of a needle. Biofeedback can determine symptoms of stress, and through training, alleviate these symptoms.

Bio-feedback may be used to improve health, performance, and the physiological changes that often occur in conjunction with changes to thoughts, emotions, and behavior. Eventually, these changes may be maintained without the use of extra equipment, as no equipment is necessarily required to practice biofeedback.

Neurofeedback (EEG feedback) is the voluntary regulation of brain wave activity. It is a learned response, with applications including the modulation of arousal levels, regulating sleep/wake cycles, dealing with cognitive processes, processing sensory information, correcting inappropriate motor responses, controlling moods and emotions, and helping deal with memory issues. This method may be helpful for PTSD and complex PTSD and may take up to 30 sessions for total results.

BRAINSPOTTING

Brainspotting is a focused treatment method that grew out of EMDR. (EMDR, also known as rapid eye movement, is discussed in depth a few chapters later in this psychological section. Brainspotting works by identifying, processing, and releasing core neurophysiological sources of emotional/body pain, trauma, dissociation, and a variety of other challenging symptoms. Brainspotting is a simultaneous form of diagnosis and treatment.

Brainspotting is a tool to neuro-biologically locate, focus, process, and release experiences and symptoms that are typically out of reach of the conscious mind and its cognitive and language capacity.

Brainspotting works with the deep brain and the body through its direct access to the autonomic and limbic systems within the body's central nervous system. Brainspotting theoretically taps into and harnesses the body's innate self-scanning capacity to process and release focused areas (systems) which are in a maladaptive, frozen, primitive survival mode.

A Brainspot is the eye position which is related to the energetic/emotional activation of a traumatic/emotionally charged issue within the brain, most likely in the amygdala, the hippocampus, or the orbitofrontal cortex of the limbic system. Located by eye position, paired with externally observed and internally experienced reflexive responses, a Brainspot is actually a physiological subsystem holding emotional experience in memory form. Brainspotting appears to stimulate, focus, and activate the body's inherent capacity to heal itself from trauma.

Brainspotting can also locate and strengthen mental resources such as clarity and creativity using the brain's extraordinary power. Brainspotting dismantles the trauma, symptom, somatic distress, and dysfunctional beliefs at the reflexive core. Everything is aimed at activating, locating, and processing the Brainspot.

Brainspotting is most powerful and effective when done with the enhancement of BioLateral Sound CDs.

Any life event which causes significant physical and/or emotional injury and distress, in which the person powerfully experiences being overwhelmed, helpless, or trapped, can become a traumatic experience. There is growing recognition within the healing professions that experiences of physical and/or emotional injury, acute and chronic pain, serious physical illness, dealing with difficult medical interventions, societal turmoil, environmental disaster, and other problematic life events, will contribute to the development of life trauma.

Medical and psychological literature now acknowledges that approximately 75% of requests for medical care are linked to the actions or consequences of this accumulation of stress and/or trauma upon the systems of the human body. Traumatic life experiences, whether physical or emotional, are often significant contributing factors in the development and/or maintenance of most of the symptoms and problems encountered in health care.

COMPLEX PTSD THERAPY

Single traumatic events like car accidents or natural disasters usually only last a short interval of minutes, hours or days. But some people experience chronic trauma that continues or repeats for months, years, even decades. This chronic trauma is known as complex post-traumatic stress disorder. Complex PTSD is not yet listed in the current Diagnostic and Statistical Manual of Mental Disorders (DSM) that is widely referred to by psychologists, psychiatrists, physicians, and insurance companies.

People who experience chronic trauma often report additional symptoms along with formal PTSD symptoms, such as changes in their self-concept and the way they adapt to stressful events including isolation and dysfunctional emotional and relationship responses.

Dr. Judith Herman of Harvard University suggests that a new diagnosis, Complex PTSD, is needed to describe the symptoms of long-term trauma.

Another name sometimes used to describe the cluster of symptoms referred to as Complex PTSD is Disorders of Extreme Stress Not Otherwise Specified (DESNOS). A work group has also proposed a diagnosis of Developmental Trauma Disorder (DTD) for children and adolescents who experience chronic traumatic events. Traumatic memories stay stuck in the brain's non-verbal, non-conscious, subcortical regions (amygdala, thalamus, hippocampus, hypothalamus, and brain stem). Those memories are not accessible to the frontal lobes—the understanding, thinking, reasoning parts of the brain. The paradox at the heart of this trauma is that survivors see and feel only their trauma, or they see and feel nothing at all, while the emotional mind believes and acts as if that the trauma is still happening.

Because results from the DSM-IV Field Trials indicated that 92% of individuals with Complex PTSD/DESNOS also met diagnostic criteria for PTSD, complex PTSD was not added as a separate diagnosis classification. However, cases that involve prolonged, repeated trauma may indicate a need for special treatment considerations. Examples of such traumatic situations include:

- long-term childhood physical abuse and abandonment
- long-term childhood sexual abuse
- long-term domestic violence
- organized child exploitation rings
- concentration camps
- prisoner of war camps
- prostitution brothels

Standard evidence-based treatments for PTSD are effective for treating PTSD. However, treating Complex PTSD often involves addressing interpersonal difficulties and specific symptoms. Dr. Herman contends that recovery from Complex PTSD requires restoration of control and power for the traumatized person. Survivors can become empowered by healing relationships which create safety, allow for remembrance and mourning, and promote reconnection with everyday life.

Because C-PTSD is a relatively new recognized condition, there's still some debate about how it should be treated. Exposure therapy, which is highly effective with PTSD, tends not to work with C-PTSD because there may be dozens of traumatic memories over years or even decades of trauma, so exposure therapy is impractical. Instead, C-PTSD researchers (Judith Herman, Bessel van der Kolk, Pete Walker, Mary Beth Williams, and Soili Poijula) generally recommend a stage-based treatment approach that includes the following phases:

- establishing safety and helping the client find ways to feel safe in his or her environment or eliminate dangers in the environment
- teaching basic self-regulation skills
- identifying and working through emotional flashbacks
- deconstructing the inner critic
- encouraging information processing that builds introspection
- helping the client to integrate his or her traumatic experiences
- encouraging healthy relationships and engagement
- strategies designed to reduce distress and increase positive affect

EMDR, Brainspotting, and Neurofeedback are all methods thought to be helpful in treating PTSD and complex PTSD.

Neurofeedback (EEG feedback) is the voluntary regulation of brain wave activity. It is a learned response, with applications including the modulation of arousal levels, regulating sleep/wake cycles, dealing with cognitive processes, processing sensory information, correcting inappropriate motor responses, controlling moods and emotions, and helping deal with memory issues. This method may be helpful for PTSD and complex PTSD and may take up to 30 sessions for total results.

A new therapy using MDMA combined with intensive counseling is currently undergoing clinical trials. MDMA is a high quality, pharmaceutical grade of the drug commonly known as Ecstasy. Researchers are investigating whether a few low doses of MDMA may assist in treating severe, treatment-resistant post-traumatic stress disorder (PTSD). In November 2016, phase 3 clinical trials for PTSD were approved by the United States Food and Drug Administration to assess effectiveness and safety and may be available to the public in 2022. This treatment is believed to eradicate the life-damaging effects of PTSD and complex PTSD.

COGNITIVE THERAPY

Cognitive therapy (CT) is a type of psychotherapy developed by American psychiatrist Aaron T. Beck. CT is one of the therapeutic approaches within the larger group of cognitive behavioral therapies (CBT) and was first expounded by Beck in the 1960s. Cognitive therapy is based on the cognitive model, which states that thoughts, feelings, and behavior are all connected, and that individuals can move toward overcoming difficulties and meeting their goals by identifying and changing unhelpful or inaccurate thinking, problematic behavior, and distressing emotional responses. This involves the individual working collaboratively with the therapist to develop skills for testing and modifying beliefs, identifying distorted thinking, relating to others in different ways, and changing behaviors. A tailored cognitive case conceptualization is developed by the cognitive therapist as a roadmap to understand the individual's internal reality, to select appropriate interventions and identify areas of distress.

Beck became disillusioned with long-term psychodynamic approaches based on gaining insight into unconscious emotions and drives, and came to the conclusion that the way in which his clients perceived, interpreted, and attributed meaning in their daily lives—a process scientifically known as cognition—was a key to therapy. Albert Ellis had been working on similar ideas since the 1950s. He called his approach Rational Therapy (RT) at first, then Rational Emotive Therapy (RET) and later Rational Emotive Behavior Therapy (REBT).

Beck outlined his approach in Depression: Causes and Treatment in 1967. He later expanded his focus to include anxiety disorders, and other disorders and problems in Cognitive Therapy and the Emotional Disorders in 1976. He also introduced a focus on the fundamental underlying ways in which people process information about the self, the world, or the future.

The new cognitive approach came into conflict with the behaviorism therapy popular at the time, which denied that talk of mental causes was scientific or meaningful, rather than simply assessing stimuli and behavioral responses.

The 1970s saw a general cognitive revolution in psychology. Behavioral modification techniques and cognitive therapy techniques became joined together, giving rise to cognitive behavioral therapy. Precursors of certain fundamental aspects of cognitive therapy have been identified in various ancient philosophical traditions, particularly Stoicism. Beck believed that the philosophical origins of cognitive therapy can be traced back to the Stoic philosophers of Greece.

EMDR—EYE MOVEMENT DESENSITIZATION AND REPROCESSING

Eye movement desensitization and reprocessing (EMDR) has grown in popularity, particularly for treating post-traumatic stress disorder (PTSD). PTSD often occurs after experiences such as military combat, physical assault, rape, or car accidents.

EMDR approaches psychological issues in an unusual way. EMDR does not rely on talk therapy or medications. Instead, EMDR uses a patient's own rapid, rhythmic eye movements to access the past trauma. These eye movements dampen the power of emotionally charged memories of past traumatic events.

An EMDR treatment session can last up to 90 minutes. The therapist will move his or her fingers back and forth in front of the client's face and ask him/her to follow these hand motions with his/her eyes. At the same time, the EMDR therapist will have the client recall a disturbing event. This will include the emotions and body sensations accompany it.

Gradually, the therapist will guide the patient to shift thoughts to more pleasant ones. Some therapists use alternatives to finger movements, such as hand or toe tapping or musical tones. Before and after each EMDR treatment, the therapist will ask a client to rate his/her level of distress. The hope is that disturbing memories will become less disabling.

EMDR is used to treat psychological problems including:
- PTSD and complex PTSD
- panic attacks
- eating disorders
- addictions

- anxiety, such as discomfort with public speaking or dental procedures phobias.

EMOTIONAL FREEDOM TECHNIQUE

Emotional Freedom Techniques (EFT) is a self-help method reducing the emotional trauma which contributes greatly to disease. EFT uses elements of Cognitive Therapy and Exposure Therapy, and combines them with Acupressure, in the form of fingertip tapping on 12 acupuncture points. Over 100 papers published in peer-reviewed medical and psychology journals, including dozens of clinical trials, have demonstrated that EFT is effective for phobias, anxiety, depression, posttraumatic stress disorder, pain, and other problems.

Clinical trials have shown that EFT tapping is able to rapidly reduce the emotional impact of memories and incidents that trigger emotional distress. Once the distress is reduced or removed, the body can often rebalance itself, and healing is accelerated.

GESTALT

Gestalt psychology (meaning shape or form in German) is a philosophy of mind of the Berlin School of experimental psychology. Gestalt psychology attempts to understand an apparently chaotic world and to help an individual make sense of it.

The central principle of Gestalt psychology is that the mind forms a comprehensive whole with self-organizing tendencies. This principle, according to Gestalt psychologist Kurt Koffka, maintains that when the human mind forms a precept or gestalt, the whole has a reality of its own, independent of the parts.

In the study of perception, Gestalt psychologists explain that perceptions are the products of complex interactions among various stimuli. Contrary to the behaviorist approach to focusing on stimulus and response, gestalt psychologists seek to understand the organization of cognitive processes. The gestalt effect is the capability of our brain to generate whole forms, particularly with respect to the visual recognition of global figures instead of just collections of simpler and unrelated elements of points, lines, and curves.

HYPNOSIS

Hypnosis is a state of human consciousness involving focused attention and reduced peripheral awareness and an enhanced capacity to respond to suggestion. The term may also refer to an art, skill, or act of inducing hypnosis.

Theories explaining what occurs during hypnosis fall into two groups. Altered state theories see hypnosis as an altered state of mind or trance, marked by a level of awareness different from the ordinary conscious state. In contrast, non-state theories see hypnosis as a form of imaginative role-enactment.

During hypnosis, a person is said to have heightened focus and concentration. The person can concentrate intensely on a specific thought or memory, while blocking out sources of distraction. Hypnotized subjects show an increased response to suggestions. Hypnosis is usually induced by a procedure known as a hypnotic induction involving a series of preliminary instructions and suggestion. The use of hypnotism for therapeutic purposes is referred to as hypnotherapy and is helpful for eating disorders, smoking cessation, and recalling troubling memories.

NEURO-LINGUISTIC PROGRAMMING (NLP)

Neuro-linguistic programing (NLP) is an approach to communication, personal development, and psychotherapy created by Richard Bandler and John Grinder in the 1970s. NLP's creators claim there is a connection between neurological processes (neuro-), language (linguistic) and behavioral patterns learned through experience (programming), and that these can be changed to achieve specific goals in life. NLP methodology can model the skills of exceptional people, allowing anyone to acquire those skills.

Neuro-Linguistic Programming was specifically created in order to allow people to create new ways of understanding how verbal and non-verbal communication affect the human brain. NLP presents everyone with the opportunity to not only communicate better with others, but also learn how to gain more control over what was considered to be automatic functions of human neurology.

Neuro-Linguistic Programming is like a user's manual for the brain, and taking an NLP training is like learning how to become fluent in the language of your mind so that the unconscious will finally understand what you actually want out of life.

NLP is the study of excellent communication—both with yourself and with others. NLP was developed by modeling excellent communicators and therapists. NLP is a set of tools and techniques, but it is so much more than that. It is an attitude and a methodology of knowing how to achieve your goals and get results.

PAST LIVES THERAPY

Through past life therapy, one can enrich the experience of one's current life in a variety of ways, such as:

- unlocking difficult relationship dynamics
- resolving physical and emotional issues
- opening one's experience to the eternal nature of existence
- accessing higher spiritual knowledge and guide one's life direction.

In past life therapy the patient regresses to the source of issues and concerns based in prior life experiences. The work is based upon the premise that we are eternal beings or souls who carry forward learning and experiences from one human lifetime to another. As eternal souls, we experience physical life on Earth in a series of human bodies and associated personalities. On a soul level, we choose each life circumstance as a means of challenging ourselves with new situations and opportunities for learning.

A belief in reincarnation is not necessary for this approach to be successful. The stories and symbolic metaphors for one's real-life issues and situations are illuminating. Past lives therapy helps people resolve issues and get past impediments and obstructions that were resistant to other therapeutic methods and to understand one's personality in greater depth.

My book *Traveling on the River of Time* (2017) is a self-help, stress-free, and trauma-free handbook intended to assist in one's own past lives therapy.

PRIMAL THERAPY

Primal therapy is a trauma-based psychotherapy created by Dr. Arthur Janov, who theorizes that neurosis is caused by the repressed pain of childhood trauma. Repressed pain can be sequentially brought to conscious awareness and resolved through re-experiencing specific incidents and fully expressing the resulting pain during therapy. In therapy, the patient recalls and reenacts particularly disturbing past experiences usually occurring early in life and expresses normally repressed anger or frustration especially through spontaneous and unrestrained screams, hysteria, or violence.

Primal therapy was developed as a means of eliciting repressed pain in order to release it. The term "pain" is used in discussions of primal therapy when referring to any repressed emotional distress and its long-lasting psychological effects. Primal therapy goes deeper than talking therapies, as those deal primarily with the cerebral cortex and higher-reasoning areas and do not access the source of pain within the more basic, primal parts of the central nervous system.

Primal therapy is used to re-experience childhood pain—i.e., felt rather than conceptual memories—in an attempt to resolve the pain through complete processing and integration. An intended objective of the therapy is to lessen or eliminate the early trauma and reduce its influence or damage to adult behavior.

Primal therapy examines the power of beliefs and how they are used as a mechanism for dealing with early trauma that can go as far back as birth or even pregnancy. Beliefs can be used to rationalize pain rooted deep in the unconscious.

PTSD THERAPY

Post-traumatic stress disorder (PTSD) is a form of anxiety that some people develop after witnessing or experiencing a traumatic event or series of events, such as warfare, rape, violence, car accident, or an incident such as 9/11. The symptoms of PTSD include nightmares, flashbacks, severe distress, and social isolation. Finding a therapist and/or a therapeutic group you trust is important. A suitable therapist will listen to your concerns and help you make changes in your life.

Many types of treatment for PTSD are available. Treatment can help you feel more in control of your emotions and result in fewer symptoms, but you may still have some bad memories. Counseling may include a therapist on your own or in a group dealing with the traumatic event and

PTSD. You will talk with your therapist and group members about your memories and feelings. This will help you change how you think about your trauma. You will learn how to deal with painful feelings and memories, so you can feel better.

Several types of counseling and therapy have been shown to be effective:

- cognitive therapy, in which the client learns to change thoughts about the trauma that are not true or that cause stress
- exposure therapy, in which the client talks about the traumatic event over and over, in a safe place, until the client has less fear
- EMDR and Brainspotting
- EEG Neurofeedback—the voluntary regulation of brain wave activity. It is a learning method with applications including the modulation of arousal levels, regulating sleep/wake cycles, dealing with cognitive processes, processing sensory information, correcting inappropriate motor responses, controlling moods and emotions, and helping deal with memory issues. This method may be helpful for PTSD and complex PTSD, and may take up to 30 sessions for full results.

A new therapy using MDMA, a high-quality, pharmaceutical grade of the drug known as Ecstasy, combined with intensive counseling, is currently undergoing clinical trials. Researchers are investigating whether a few low doses of MDMA may help in treating severe, treatment-resistant posttraumatic stress disorder (PTSD). In November 2016, phase three clinical trials for PTSD were approved by the United States Food and Drug Administration to assess effectiveness and safety. This therapy may be available to the public by 2022. This treatment is believed to eradicate the life-damaging effects of PTSD and complex PTSD.

REDECISION THERAPY

Redecision therapy is based on the assumption that adults made decisions based on messages absorbed in childhood from their parents and caretakers. These messages, along with other evaluations, inform current decision-making processes, which can have negative effects.

In Redecision therapy, individuals can examine these messages and any past negative decisions in order to identify what is not working. With the help of a therapist, people in therapy may be able to adopt new meanings and extinguish self-defeating decision-making patterns through the use of reflective exploration and experiential techniques.

This therapy, developed in 1965 by social worker Mary Goulding and her husband, psychiatrist Bob Goulding, combines the theoretical framework of Transactional Analysis with the interventional techniques of Gestalt therapy. Dissatisfied with the therapeutic frameworks of the day, the Gouldings sought to create a modality that was brief and effective and thus developed a fusion of both models, recognizing the way each model complemented the objective of the other.

The ultimate goal of Redecision therapy is for a patient to review all choices and decisions made that might influence a current problem or situation. This type of therapy is often able to help individuals isolate negative implications attached to a situation and learn how to release the emotions and messages attached to them. Past experiences are not overly examined, but they are considered to be a vital component in the facilitation of changes toward behavior that can result in a more positive sense of well-being.

The therapist works to help the patient create new messages and beliefs, encouraging the person in therapy to recognize and strengthen aspects of the true self.

Throughout treatment, first-person narratives are explored, and in these, an individual may use language and emotion to describe situations that are currently occurring and, with the help of the therapist, identify and explore ways that past experiences are being replayed in current relationships. One may untangle the meanings and implications of the messages, called injunctions (such as don't think, don't enjoy, don't feel, don't exist, don't grow up, etc.), in order to improve the way one interacts with the world.

Some examples of Redecision therapy techniques include the following:

the empty chair: The person in therapy chooses a scene to reenact, usually an early scene involving a parent, and then conducts a dialogue with the parent. The therapist acts as a director, supporting the individual in adapting the scene to include new conversations and choices that contribute to current goals.

- **Early scene work:** The person in therapy replays a scene from childhood, reliving the memory. The therapist asks the child persona questions related to thoughts, feelings, and choices made. One goal of this exercise is to determine how these scenes resulted in beliefs and decisions that are currently keeping the person stuck.
- **The parent interview:** The therapist asks the person in therapy to impersonate a parent. The therapist then interviews the "parent," asking about life experiences, feelings, and decisions. One goal of this exercise is to gain insight into the parent's point of view.
- **Dream work:** If the person in therapy had a dream that ended badly or was interrupted, the therapist can help the individual rework the ending in a positive way.

REICHIAN THERAPY

Reichian therapy can refer to several schools of thought and therapeutic techniques whose common touchstone is their origin in the work of psychoanalyst Wilhelm Reich (1897–1957). Some examples are:

- Bioenergetic analysis, which combines psychological analysis, active work with the body, and relational therapeutic work.
- Body psychotherapy, which addresses the body and the mind as a whole with emphasis on the reciprocal relationships within body and mind.
- Neo-Reichian massage, whose practitioners attempt to locate and dissolve body armoring (also called "holding patterns").
- Vegetotherapy, a form of psychotherapy that involves the physical manifestations of emotions.

(also see Bodywork—Reichian therapy)

SENSORY DEPRIVATION

Sensory deprivation (Sendep) or isolation is the deliberate reduction or removal of stimuli from one or more of the senses. Simple devices such as blindfolds, hoods, or earmuffs can cut off sight and hearing, while more complex devices can also cut off the sense of smell, touch, taste, thermoception (heat sensing), and gravity.

Sensory deprivation has been used in various alternative health care and in psychological experiments. Short term sessions of sensory deprivation are described as relaxing and conducive to meditation.

A related phenomenon is perceptual deprivation, also called the ganzfeld effect. In this case a constant uniform stimulus is used instead of attempting to remove the stimuli, which leads to effects which have similarities to sensory deprivation.

In chamber REST, the subject lies on a bed in a completely dark and sound-reducing (on average, 80 dB) room for up to 24 hours. Their movement is restricted by the experimental instructions, but not by any mechanical restraints. Food, drin,k and toilet facilities are provided in the room and are at the discretion of the tester. Subjects are allowed to leave the room before the 24 hours are complete; however, fewer than 10% actually do.

In flotation REST, the room contains a tank or pool. The flotation medium consists of a skin-temperature solution of water and Epsom salts at a specific gravity that allows for the patient to float supine without worry of safety. In fact, to turn over while in the solution requires major deliberate effort. Fewer than 5% of the subjects tested leave before the session duration ends, which is usually around an hour for flotation REST. For the first 40 minutes, it is reportedly possible to experience itching in various parts of the body (a phenomenon also reported to be common during the early stages of meditation). The last 20 minutes often end with a transition from beta or alpha brainwaves to theta, which typically occur briefly before sleep and again at waking. In a float tank, the theta state can last for several minutes without the subject losing consciousness. Some use the extended theta state as a tool for enhanced creativity and problem solving. Spas sometimes provide commercial float tanks for use in relaxation. Flotation therapy has been academically studied in the U.S. and in Sweden with published results showing reductions of both pain and stress. The relaxed state also involves lowered blood pressure and maximal blood flow and sometimes smoking cessation.

Several differences exist between flotation and chamber REST. For example, with the presence of a medium in flotation REST, the subject has reduced tactile stimulation while experiencing weightlessness. The addition of Epsom salts to attain the desired specific gravity may have a therapeutic effect on tight muscles. Since one of the main effects of chamber REST is the resulting state of relaxation, the effects of chamber REST on arousal are less clear-cut, which can be attributed to the nature of the solution.

Also, due to the inherent immobilization that is experienced in flotation REST (by not being able to roll over), which can become uncomfortable after several hours, the subject is unable to experience the lengthy session durations of chamber REST. This may not allow the subject to experience the changes in attitudes and thinking that are associated with chamber REST.

Practitioners in chamber REST area have explored its utility in the treatment of major psychiatric dysfunctions such as autism and substance abuse. Flotation REST was tested more for its use with stress-related disorders, pain reduction, and insomnia.

SILVA METHOD (SILVA MIND CONTROL)

José Silva was an electrical repairman who developed a great interest in religion, psychology, and parapsychology. He spent much time learning hypnosis in an attempt to increase his children's IQ. After experimenting and being convinced of his daughter's sudden clairvoyance, Silva decided to learn more about the development of psychic abilities.

In 1944, Silva began developing his method, formerly known as Silva Mind Control, in the 1940s, using it on his family members and friends, before launching it commercially in the 1960s. Silva did research on the brain, based on Robert Sperry's split-brain theory, to improve his method. One hypothesis as to why Silva's method produced results is that he was training left-brain minds to think with their right brain.

The technique aims to reach and sustain a state of mental functioning, called alpha state, where brainwave frequency is seven to fourteen Hz. Daydreaming and the transition to sleeping are alpha states.

Silva developed a program that trained people to enter certain brain states of enhanced awareness. He developed several systematic mental processes to use while in these states allowing a person to mentally project with a specific intent. According to Silva, once the mind is projected, a person can view distant objects or locations and connect with higher intelligence for guidance. The information received by the projected mind is then said to be perceived as thoughts, images, feelings, smells, tastes, and sound by the mind. The information obtained in this manner can be acted upon to solve problems.

SOMATIC THERAPY

Our bodies are miracles of healing and are designed to self-heal. By supporting the patient through the exploration and expression of these deeper understandings, Somatic Psychotherapy can facilitate this healing. Somatic or Body Oriented Psychotherapy encourages the communication of experience between the mind and the body. This interaction allows greater understanding of the issues and enables sustainable movement towards improved health and wellbeing.

With this greater insight comes aliveness, creativity, self-regulation, and self-awareness. This perception enables the patient to deepen and strengthen personal relationships with others.

Somatic psychology is a form of alternative medicine that focuses on somatic experience and the embodied self, including therapeutic and holistic approaches to body. Body psychotherapy is a general branch of this subject, while somatherapy, eco-somatics and dance therapy, for example, are specific branches of the subject. Somatic psychology is a framework that seeks to bridge the mind-body dichotomy.

Pierre Janet can be considered the first somatic psychologist due to his extensive psychotherapeutic studies and writings with significant reference to the body, some of which pre-date Freud. It is only gradually that the body entered into the realm of available techniques that could be used in a psychodynamic frame, following the explorations of Sándor Ferenczi and his friend Georg Groddeck, then Otto Fenichel and his friend Wilhelm Reich.

Reich was the first to try to develop a clear psychodynamic approach that included the body. He then developed his own way of combining body and mind and the somatic regulators that connect these two dimensions. Reich had a significant influence in the founding of body psychotherapy (or somatic psychology as it is often known in the USA and Australia)—

though he called his early work character analysis and character-analytic vegetotherapy. Several types of body-oriented psychotherapies trace their origins back to Reich. In addition to Reichian therapy, other subsequent methods helpful in trauma work have arisen from somatic psychology.

Dance therapy, or dance movement psychotherapy, also reflects this approach and is considered a study and practice within the field of somatic psychology.

STRESS MANAGEMENT

Stress management refers to the wide spectrum of techniques and psychotherapies aimed at controlling a person's levels of stress, especially chronic stress, for the purpose of improving everyday functioning. In this context, the term stress refers to significant negative consequences, or distress in the terminology advocated by Hans Selye, rather than what he calls eustress, a stress whose consequences are helpful or otherwise positive.

Stress produces numerous physical and mental symptoms which vary according to each individual's situational factors. These can include the decline of physical health as well as depression, anxiety, and other psychological and physiological upsets. The process of stress management is one of the keys to a happy and successful life in modern society. Although life provides numerous demands that can prove difficult to handle, stress management provides a number of ways to manage anxiety and maintain overall well-being.

Despite stress often being thought of as a subjective experience, levels of stress are readily measurable using various physiological tests similar to those used in polygraphs.

Many practical stress management techniques are available, some for use by health professionals and others for self-help, which may help an individual to reduce their levels of stress, provide positive feelings of control over one's life, and promote general well-being. Evaluating the effectiveness of various stress management techniques can be difficult, as research currently exists. Consequently, the amount and quality of evidence for the various techniques varies widely. Some are accepted as effective treatments for use in traditional psychotherapy, while others with less evidence favoring them are considered alternative therapies. Many professional organizations exist to promote and provide training in conventional or alternative therapies.

Acute stress is the most common form of stress among humans worldwide. Acute stress deals with the pressures of the near future or dealing with the very recent past. This type of stress is often misinterpreted for being a negative connotation. While this is the case in some circumstances, it is also a good thing to have some acute stress in life. Running or any other form of exercise is considered an acute stressor. An exciting or exhilarating experience such as riding a roller coaster is an acute stress but is usually very enjoyable. Acute stress is a short-term stress and, as a result, does not have enough time to do the damage that long-term stress causes.

Chronic stress is unlike acute stress. It has a wearing effect on people that can result in a serious health risk if it continues over a long period of time. Chronic stress can lead to memory loss, damage spatial recognition, and produce a decreased drive of eating. The severity varies from person to person and gender difference can also be an underlying factor. Women are able to tolerate longer durations of stress than men without showing the same maladaptive changes. Men can deal with shorter stress duration better than women can but once males hit a certain threshold, the chances of them developing mental issues increases drastically. Some of the following methods reduce low levels of stress, while others deal with the stressor at a higher level:

Autogenic training	Social activity
Cognitive therapy	Conflict resolution
Cranial release technique	Getting a hobby
Meditation	Mindfulness
Music as a coping strategy	Deep breathing
Yoga Nidra	Nootropics
Reading novels	Prayer
Relaxation techniques	Artistic expression
Fractional relaxation	Humor
Physical exercise	Progressive relaxation
Spas	Somatics training

Spending time in nature

Natural medicine

Planning and decision making

Listening to certain types of
relaxing music

Clinically validated alternative
treatments

Stress balls

Time management

Spending quality time with pets

TWELVE-STEP PROGRAMS

Twelve-Step programs are well known for their use in recovering from addictive and dysfunctional behaviors. The first 12-step program began with Alcoholics Anonymous (A.A.) in the 1930s and has since grown to be the most widely used approach in dealing not only with recovery from alcoholism, but also from drug abuse as well as other addictive, compulsive, and dysfunctional behaviors.

The first book written to cover the 12-step program was titled Alcoholics Anonymous, known as the Big Book by program members. Following the subsequent extensive growth of 12-step programs for other addictive and dysfunctional behaviors, many additional books were written and recordings and videos were produced. These cover the 12 steps in greater detail and how people in recovery have specifically applied the steps in their lives. An extensive chronology and background about the history of A.A. has been put together at Dick B.'s website.

Each program follows 12 steps to recover. Groups other than A.A. who have adopted the 12 steps to address their own particular addictive or dysfunctional behavior have similar ideas, usually with only minor variations. These steps are meant to be worked sequentially as a process for getting rid of addictive behaviors and the intended result is a growth in freedom and happiness, as outlined in the Promises. The general governing approach for A.A. groups was originally laid out in the Twelve Traditions, and they remain the guiding principles for most 12- step groups today.

A wealth of information about 12 Step programs can be found on the internet, including lists of various 12-step groups located in your area.

VISUALIZATION

Creative visualization is a mental technique that uses the imagination to make dreams and goals come true. Used in the right way, creative visualization can improve your life and attract to you success and prosperity. Creative visualization is a power that can alter one's environment and circumstances, cause events to happen, and attract money, possessions, work, people, and love into your life.

Creative visualization uses the power of the mind, and is the power behind every success. By visualizing a certain event, situation, or an object, it can be attracted into one's life, through a process similar to daydreaming. Although this might seem like magic, there is no magic involved, only the natural process of the power of thoughts and natural mental laws.

Some people use this technique naturally in their everyday affairs, not being aware that they are using a sort of personal power. All successful people use it consciously or unconsciously, to attract the success they want into their life by visualizing their goals as already accomplished.

The subconscious mind accepts thoughts that are repeated often. When it accepts them, it changes one's mindset accordingly, as well as habits and actions. This new and improved mindset brings one into contact with new people, situations, and circumstances.

Thoughts are endowed with a creative power that molds one's life, and attracts what is thought about. Thoughts travel from one mind to another, and if they are strong enough, they can be unconsciously picked up by other people who are in a position to help achieve one's desires and goals.

Thoughts can come true. Not all your thoughts, but those that are focused, well-defined, and often-repeated.

Thought is energy, especially a focused thought, soaked with emotional energy. Thoughts change the balance of energy around us, and bring changes to the environment in accordance with them.

Most people think and repeat certain thoughts quite often. Focusing thoughts on their current environment and situation will create and recreate those events and circumstances, whether it is worrying or concentrating on a specific positive outcome.

"The Universal Bank Account" and "How to Get What You Want" are two essays in my book *Cosmic Grandma Wisdom* about utilizing creative visualization with concrete steps to success.

HEALTH PRODUCTS

An important adjunct to alternative health care and therapies are various health products. I have included some of the products available on the market, ones that my family and I have tested, as well as testimonials from friends and health professionals.

Sometimes a particular product has been an essential key when incorporated into someone's health regimen. Health products can be an integral part of a particular therapy. For example, supplements are used in holistic and alternative health care, while soy products are an important element of Macrobiotics.

Herbs and vitamins/supplements are an extensive study and could be several books unto themselves.

ALOE VERA

Aloe Vera is a plant from the lily family. The gel and juice from three-year old outer leaves is extracted for a variety of uses and for many ailments. It is taken internally as a juice, and externally as a rub, a poultice, a skin cleanser, and a salve. These products must be properly stabilized, which ensures that the useful elements in the fresh gel have been successfully preserved.

Aloe Vera is considered a food and contains magnesium, zinc, sodium, potassium, chlorine, calcium, copper, and chromium.

Its uses, according to recent studies, are numerous:
- eye wash, good for eye infections
- used against herpes simplex and herpes zoster

- helpful as a mouthwash for periodontal surgery, tooth or gum pain, or as a gel applied to a surgical wound
- insect bites, poison ivy, and poison oak
- effective in treating ventricular ulcers, diverticulitis, lung deposits, sinusitis, monilial infections, trichomonas,
- scleroderma, pyorrhea, clouded cornea, and snakebite
- as a douche against candida albicans
- for external use on eczema, abrasions, cuts, burns, windburn, chafing, sunburn, athlete's foot, fever blisters, joint and muscle pain

Aloe Vera is used on professional athletes to treat their injuries at the University of Texas, the Dallas Cowboys, and the Baltimore Colts. Injuries heal quicker with Aloe Vera than using traditional treatment, according to Spanky Stevens, former head trainer for the University of Texas. Injuries being treated are: strains, sprains, bruises, cramps, swelling, soreness, pain in muscles, tendons, and joints, inflammation and skin irritations, itching, turf burns, blisters, fungus, skin infections, sunburn, bursitis, and tendonitis. In addition, Aloe Vera can be used to treat sick and injured animals such as cats, dogs, horses, and cows.

Aloe Vera is not new. It was used extensively in ancient times. In the past 30 years, the medical properties of Aloe Vera have been rediscovered and analyzed. Aloe has been approved by the U.S. Food and Drug Administration (FDA) as a safe food additive.

P.S. A woman I knew in Sacramento was very ill and had been tested for hypoglycemia. She had such severe low blood sugar that even being administered the glucose tolerance test affected her adversely. During most of the two years that I knew her, she went to a nutritionist, an herbalist, a reflexologist, and some other alternative health care practitioners. Her health continued to deteriorate and she was forced to quit her job and live on disability payments and savings. Then someone recommended that she try drinking Aloe Vera juice, which she did. Within a week her health had dramatically improved, her energy increased, even the color in her face became rosy. She started looking and acting like a completely different person than when I had met her. She became an Aloe Vera distributor to share her discovery with other ill people. It was due to her amazing progress that I became interested in Aloe Vera.

BIRKENSTOCK SHOES

The foot was made for movement over natural ground that would yield, thereby supporting the whole foot. The bones and tissues within feet are best adapted to this environment. Also, the human body is meant to work in an upright position, with the heel resting at the same elevation as the ball of the foot. On a healthy foot the big and little toes line up with the sides of the foot, but modern shoes squeeze the toes into a too-narrow space. Modern footwear generally has elevated heels which throws body posture off. Fatigue, nosebleeds, backaches, headaches, and leg cramps can result over time wearing modern shoes.

Doctors tell us that inactivity has caused much of our population to become overweight. When overweight bodies are supported by fashion shoes with high heels, or even with low heels, the bodyweight is redistributed onto the toes which are squeezed too tightly into the shoes to move. Our bodies depend on the movement of our toes to help our blood circulate. Toes are motors that power your leg muscles, which are sometimes called your second heart. When you walk, your leg muscles help your first heart by pumping blood back up through the veins.

That's why walking can be so helpful in keeping your heart healthy. When you walk in Birkenstock shoes, your toes can always move freely, and everything else can work the way it was designed to work.

Birkenstock sandals and shoes are the result of years of study about the human body. Birkenstock shoes allows the foot to function naturally. Birkenstock sandals recreate that barefoot-on-the-beach feeling, and contribute to a healthier, more natural walk. The front of the sandal allows plenty of room for the toes. The heel rests in a normal position within a cradling heel cup for stability and support. The foot bed is made so that it remolds to accommodate the shape of the arch.

These shoes are recommended for people with heel pain symptoms due to rheumatoid arthritis, ankylosing spondylitis, systemic lupus erythematosus, heel spurs, gouty arthritis, and plantar fasciitis. These symptoms can be alleviated or greatly relieved by the regular wearing of Birkenstock sandals, after the initial remolding period. Many diabetics can benefit from wearing Birkenstock shoes (get your doctor's okay first).

You do not have to have foot problems or pain to enjoy Birkenstock shoes or sandals. They are very comfortable to wear and have a natural look.

Because so many people are used to wearing regular shoes, the Achilles tendon shortens. Therefore, it may take time for the legs to get used to the natural posture derived from Birkenstock shoes and sandals.

For those who must wear regular footwear, Birkenstock has a variety of insoles and arch supports (orthotics) for most types of footwear, and the Birko-sport insole system can be used in athletic shoes (for preventive and corrective treatments), work boots, or shoes. Many people experience relief from foot discomfort by using these support systems. Many Birkenstock shoe dealers can take prescriptions for certain foot problems and the shoes are then especially made for the wearer.

There are other healthful footwear products on the market, but those aren't included in this book.

BONE BROTH

Bone broth is a soothing, nutrient-dense addition to the kitchen table, and wonderfully easy and inexpensive to make at home. It's extraordinarily rich in protein, specifically gelatin, and also contains trace amounts of minerals like calcium and phosphorus. Making your own bone broth from scratch is easy and economical. If you don't have the time or would rather not fuss with simmering bones for hours to make broth, you can buy excellent, traditionally prepared bone broth. I know several women diagnosed with osteoporosis who drink bone broth liberally to strengthen their bones.

Just before this book went to print, I discovered another therapeutic application of bone broth. GAPS which stands for Gut and Psychology Syndrome, is a program designed by Dr. Natasha Campbell-McBride to treat her own suffering child. GAPS is a natural nutritional treatment system for a wide variety of illnesses, ranging from various digestive problems, like leaky gut syndrome, colitis, and acid reflux, to autism, dyspraxia, A.D.D., dyslexia, A.D.H.D., depression, schizophrenia, as well as atherosclerosis, angina, heart attack, high blood pressure, stroke, arrhythmia, and peripheral vascular disease.

CMO (CETYL MYRISOLEATE)

CMO was discovered in 1972 by Harry W. Diehl, Ph.D., a researcher at the National Institutes of Health. At the time, Dr. Diehl was testing anti-inflammatory drugs on lab animals. He first artificially induced arthritis in the animals by injecting a heat-killed bacterium called Freund's adjuvant into them. Dr. Diehl discovered that Swiss albino mice did not get arthritis after the injection. Eventually he was able to determine that CMO was the factor naturally present in the mice that was responsible for the protection. When CMO was injected into various strains of rats, it offered the same protection against arthritis.

CMO protects against osteoarthritis and rheumatoid arthritis and is effective as a joint lubricant and an anti-inflammatory agent.

COLLOIDAL SILVER

"According to a report written by Richard Davies and Samuel Etris of The Silver Institute in a 1996...colloidal silver can help heal the body." https://draxe.com/colloidal-silver-benefits/

Colloidal silver attaches to ALL bacteria, kills that bacteria, and prevents the bacteria DNA from reproducing.

Benefits include:

- Anti-bacterial (apply topically)
- Wound care/skin health (apply topically)
- Pink eye/ear infections (apply topically)
- Anti-viral
- Anti-inflammatory (sip once a day for prevention)
- Sinusitis (spray into nostrils)
- Cold/flu prevention and treatment (take a sip a few times a day until symptoms abate)
- Pneumonia (take a sip a few times a day; can also be used with oxygen inhalation)

Colloidal silver can reduce the effects and recurring outbreaks of herpes viruses and Epstein Barr. When taking colloidal silver orally it is helpful to hold the liquid in the mouth for several minutes. The colloidal silver will thus be absorbed directly into the body via the salivary glands.

DIGESTIVE ENZYMES AND BETAINE HYDROCHLORIC ACID

Food is medicine. Thomas Edison is quoted as saying: "The doctor of the future will give no medicine but will interest his patients in the care of the human frame, in diet, and in the cause and prevention of disease."

Digestion is a crucial and complex function necessary to digest food. Most of the body's energy goes into digesting food.

Digestion starts in the mouth, then continues in the stomach and through the intestines. Digestion is needed to break down food so that the body can utilize the nutrients. Without proper digestion, no amount of nutrients —both from food and from supplements —can be utilized.

Enzymes are vital for digestion, without which stomach distress such as bloating, acid indigestion, stomach aches, and other problems can result. Enzymes that are secreted in the stomach are called gastric enzymes including pepsin—a total of 700 enzymes in all. The stomach plays a major role in digestion, both in a mechanical sense by mixing and crushing the food, and also in an enzymatic sense, by digesting it. Cooking food kills enzymes.

Hydrochloric acid (HCl) is stomach acid which is produced by the cells of the stomach and helps to digest proteins. HCl mainly functions to denature the proteins ingested, to destroy any bacteria or virus that remains in the food, and also to activate pepsinogen into pepsin. Without the proper amount of calcium, hydrochloric acid cannot be produced and digestion is impaired. Conversely, hydrochloric acid is vital to assimilate calcium. Too little HCL can produce comparable symptoms as having too much acid in the stomach. An alternative medical doctor can determine the difference and prescribe accordingly.

Intrinsic factor (IF) is produced by the parietal cells of the stomach. Vitamin B12 is an important vitamin that requires assistance for absorption in the terminal ileum of the small intestine. Haptocorrin is secreted by salivary glands which binds Vitamin B; its purpose is to protect Vitamin B12 from hydrochloric acid produced in the stomach. Once the stomach contents exits the stomach into the duodenum, haptocorrin is attached to pancreatic enzymes, releasing the intact vitamin B12. Intrinsic factor then binds Vitamin B12, creating a Vitamin B12-IF complex. This complex is then absorbed at the terminal portion of the ileum which intersects with the large intestine.

Mucin: The stomach has a priority to destroy bacteria and viruses using its highly acidic environment but also has a duty to protect its own lining from its acid. The way that the stomach achieves this is by secreting mucin and bicarbonate via its mucous cells, and also by having a rapid cell turnover.

Gastrin is an important hormone produced by the G cells of the stomach. G cells produce gastrin in response to stomach stretching occurring after food enters it, and also after stomach exposure to protein. Gastrin is an endocrine hormone and enters the bloodstream and eventually returns to the stomach where it stimulates parietal cells to produce hydrochloric acid and intrinsic factor.

Gastric lipase is an acidic lipase secreted by the gastric chief cells in the stomach. It has a pH optimum of 3–6. Gastric lipase and lingual lipase comprise the two acidic lipases. "These lipases, unlike alkaline lipases (such as pancreatic lipase), do not require bile acid or colipase for optimal enzymatic activity." wikipedia.com

You can discuss digestive problems with your health care practitioner, who can determine if you have too much acid in your stomach—or too little. Your practitioner may prescribe digestive enzymes and/or betaine hydrochloric acid to supplement your intake. Digestive enzymes and HCL diminish with aging, so older people often have digestive problems. Antacids and medications are regularly prescribed for digestive upset but may not help with the underlying problem.

FOOD: ORGANIC; NON-GMO; FREE RANGE MEAT AND EGGS; PASTURE RAISED MEATS AND EGGS

Not only are these foods superior for health, they are tastier and have a longer shelf-life. You can feel the nutrients as you eat.

HERBS

Herbs are the oldest form of medicine practiced by mankind. Herbs have been found at the grave site of a Neanderthal man. In 2800 BC Shen Nung, a Chinese herbalist, listed 366 plant drugs, including the one found at the prehistoric grave. The American Indians, Chinese, East Indians, and a growing number of Western cultures use herbs for healing, prevention of illness, balancing the body, anesthesia, analgesics, and contraception. Herbs also soothe, provide nourishment, and influence fertility. Herbs and plants fight major illnesses, such as cancer and heart disease, as well as help heal coughs, colds, digestive ailments, and many other complaints.

Herbal remedies are used singly or in combination with each other. Remedies utilize roots, leaves, berries, flowers, and the bark of plants. In the case of Chinese medicine, the herbs are sometimes mixed with animal and mineral extracts.

Each herb works especially well on a part of the body, and/or combats a specific ailment. Sometimes certain herbs are formulated together to join forces towards healing that ailment.

The following are ways in which herbs are prepared for use:
- **Decoction**—a tea is made of the roots and bark
- **Fomentation**—a tea is made of the leaves and blossoms
- **Oil of herbs**—an extraction of an herb is made from an oil base
- **Poultice**—a moist, hot pack applied externally and locally
- **Tincture**—an extraction of herbs in vinegar or alcohol
- **Capsules or tablets**—herbs are dried and compressed into tablets or powdered and put in capsules

Products helpful for sore, achy muscles, tendons, and ligaments, as well as for bruised, strained, and torn tissues are:
- Bruise, Strain and Tear Repair ointment
- Arnica homeopathic gels and ointments

JUICES

Raw, freshly juiced fruits and vegetables are extremely beneficial for health. They are rich in vitamins, minerals, trace elements, enzymes, and natural sugars.

Hundreds of nutrients in juice are assimilated directly into the bloodstream from the mouth and stomach. Juices are easy on the digestive system and can speed recovery from disease by supplying substances for healing. Juices provide alkaline abundance—over-acidity contributes to disease. Easily assimilated organic minerals restore balance in tissue and cells. Juices contain nature's own medicines, hormones, and antibiotics. Juices contains a factor which stimulates micro-electric tension in tissues and helps cells to absorb nutrients and expel toxins and waste. The value of raw juices is that they furnish the body with the necessary materials for body functioning and repair.

Juice should be prepared immediately before drinking. Nutrients are lost in the first 15 minutes after juicing. This is true of all juicers except for the hydraulic press juicer, which does not oxidize the fruits and vegetables. The juice from the hydraulic press can be stored for up to 48 hours with little nutritional loss.

Juice only fresh, ripe fruits, plants, berries, and vegetables, preferably organic. Wash them carefully first. Make only as much as will be drunk immediately. If juices are very sweet, they can be diluted with water 50/50. Vegetables can be mixed together. Fruits can be mixed together, except for melons which should be drunk alone. Fruit and vegetable juices do not combine well and may putrefy in the stomach. Have a juice drink between meals or one hour before meals. Avoid drinking juice with meals, as it disturbs digestion. Mix the juice in the mouth with saliva and drink slowly. More of the nutrition will be released and the digestion process will be more complete.

Fruit and vegetable juices are superior to any vitamin supplements or anything we can obtain artificially. They are easy to digest, and contain vitamins which are not yet discovered and may contain other factors, such as bioflavonoids. The miracle factor responsible in juices is dubbed Vitamin U. This factor helps to counteract the build-up of wastes from poor nutrition and stress, and speeds up the destruction of dead, diseased, or damaged cells and helps to renew the immune system.

Benefits of juices:

- Persons who have poor teeth, artificial dentures, or no teeth can take raw vegetables in form of juice.
- A person who has no time to eat a proper meal can get nourishment in the form of juice.

- A person with ulcers may have difficulty eating raw vegetables, yet he can drink carrot juice. There is no roughage to irritate, and it is very soothing, healing, and nourishing.
- A greater amount of vegetables in the form of juice can be taken into the system than could be eaten. (For example, one glass of carrot juice can be made from eight carrots. But eating eight raw carrots at one time is more difficult.)
- The raw juices are a boon to invalids who have lost their appetites.
- Raw carrot juice is excellent for little babies and growing children.
- Juices are excellent for adolescents, as they aid in the normal development of the glands and reduce pimples.
- Juices are a great aid in strengthening the aged and in preventing constipation and gall stones.
- Raw vegetable juice taken daily by young and old, healthy and ill, is a guarantee that the body is receiving its quota of building materials to heal the trillions of cells of which the body is composed.
- Juices are recommended during fasting, and can be used for weight loss and weight management.

Dr. George Lanyi, a Swedish expert on raw juice therapy who worked at the world famous Buchinger clinic in Germany for many years, claims that raw juice therapy can successfully treat heart and blood diseases, digestive disorders, rheumatism, diabetes, obesity, kidney and skin disorders, and problems such as anxiety and insomnia. A British Ministry of Health and Public Service Laboratory publication reports that juices are valuable in the relief of hypertension, cardiovascular and kidney diseases and obesity.

Raw juices beneficially treat peptic ulcers, chronic diarrhea, colitis, and toxemia. Juices are beneficial in treating excessive production of hydrochloric acid. Some experts feel that juice is a gentle treatment for cancer. It is a powerful antidote for stress and fatigue.

There are many types and models of juicers available—citrus juicers, centrifugal juicers, hydraulic press juicers, and juice extractors are but a few. The foremost expert and a legend in nutrition, juices, and juice therapy in the U.S. was Dr. Norman Walker. He researched and published books in this field for many years and there is a juicer with his name on the market.

P.S. YES, WE HAVE NO BANANAS

Years ago, I bought a Champion Juice extractor. I had low blood sugar for many years and was warned to stay away from too much fruit and fruit juices. I was impressed with the Fit for Life (food combining) authors' revolutionary stance on fruit and fruit juices. I tried eating only fruit and fresh fruit juice in the morning. My energy rocketed and my health improved immediately. Then I got totally addicted to fresh fruit juice.

Even though I may stray from eating properly the rest of the day, I do not goof up in the morning. I love juice. I find that fresh fruit juice staves off hunger until noon quite nicely and I feel wonderful. If I find my stomach is growling, I just have a little more juice. I play with combinations of many different fruits and each one is more delicious than the last. Then there are fruit smoothies, which are a million times better than milk shakes. I use fresh squeezed juice and add some fruit, like bananas, berries or papaya. For the last 40 years, I start every day with a smoothie.

Veggie juices are delectable. Although I experiment with many blends, my favorite is still good old organic carrot juice. If you have never tried it, you are in for a treat. When I drink that fabulous carrot nectar, I find that my mouth says "yum" and my body begins to "hum." I think I have become a juiceaholic.

LACTOBACILLUS ACIDOPHILUS; PROBIOTICS; PREBIOTICS

Lactobacillus acidophilus is one of many types of bacteria (probiotic) which have been shown to be beneficial in controlling the growth of certain undesirable microorganisms in the intestinal tract such as salmonella and candida albicans. In addition, according to current research, acidophilus is now found to be helpful in controlling cholesterol.

Lactobacillus acidophilus, the bacteria present in yogurt, is the predominant bacteria in the colon. This probiotic is friendly flora, a normal bacteria present in the mucous membranes, and is vital for safe-guarding health from invading bacteria and fungus. A close relationship exists between health and the kinds of bacteria found in the colon. In addition to lactobacillus acidophilus, the other types of bacteria include lactobacillus bulgaricus and lactobacillus bifidus.

Antibiotics, diabetes, birth control pills, pregnancy, and steroids are some of the things that kill off or decimate the bacteria population in the body necessary for health. Taking acidophilus orally in the form of yogurt, rejuvelac (a fermented sprouted wheat drink), in capsules, or from other sources can result in the friendly flora repopulating and establishing health in the mucous membranes. To regain normal bacterial health, lactobacillus bifidus or lactobacillus acidophilus can be implanted into the colon (by way of enemas) or vagina (by douching). Acidophilus comes in capsules, powders, and liquid form and should be refrigerated.

Many adults and children are found to have lactose intolerance (inability to digest cow's milk) and that intolerance can lead to allergic or sensitive reactions to milk. The bacteria in acidophilus has been found to supply the necessary enzyme to digest cow's milk. For those who continue to be sensitive to milk products, probiotics are also derived from soy and coconut milk as well as fermented products like sauerkraut and kambucha. I understand that food probiotics are superior to tablets or capsules. The food probiotics enable helpful bacteria to travel the entire length of the bowel.

A fairly recent nutritional treatment system called GAPS, which stands for Gut and Psychology Syndrome, uses probiotics extensively to heal multiple of health issues. GAPS is a program designed by Dr. Natasha Campbell-McBride to treat her own suffering child. GAPS is a natural treatment for a wide variety of illnesses, ranging from various digestive problems like leaky gut syndrome, colitis, and acid reflux, to autism, dyspraxia, A.D.D., dyslexia, A.D.H.D., depression, schizophrenia, as well as atherosclerosis, angina, heart attack, high blood pressure, stroke, arrhythmia, and peripheral vascular disease.

PREBIOTICS

Prebiotics are substances that induce the growth or activity of microorganisms (e.g., bacteria and fungi or probiotics) that contribute to the well-being of their host. In the diet, prebiotics are typically non-digestible fiber compounds that pass undigested through the upper part of the gastrointestinal tract and stimulate the growth or activity of advantageous bacteria that colonize the large bowel by acting as substrate for them. Prebiotics were first identified and named by Marcel Roberfroid in 1995.

LIVE FOODS

A whole carrot stored in your basement all winter can still be planted in the spring and will grow. It is a live food. But that same carrot, if cooked, is dead food, and no power on earth will make it grow.

Ripe, fresh, raw fruits and vegetables, wheatgrass and other raw juices, as well as sprouted seeds of grasses, beans, and grains are considered live food. Live foods have their nutrients intact.

Raw fruits and vegetables contain enzymes, elements which bring about necessary chemical changes in the body, which are destroyed by cooking and processing. These live foods contain in concentrated form the vitamins, minerals, trace elements, and other substances (such as chlorophyll) needed by the body. Nutrients in a single food are related to one another and cannot be replaced by the taking of single vitamins, which may upset the body's balance.

Researchers have found that substances needed for the body to utilize vitamins and minerals are found naturally in live foods. Researchers believe these substances may need to accompany vitamins and minerals into the body in order for the body to properly use the nutrients. Two such substances are bioflavonoids and hesperidin.

Live foods contain high amounts of water, essential for life. In that water resides the vitamins, minerals, enzymes, and other nutrients. Cooking removes the water and much of the nutrients. Drinking water by itself and taking vitamin tablets cannot replace what is found in fresh food.

Digestion takes more energy than any other function of the body and goes on 24 hours a day. Live food digests quickly and easily. Since the process of digestion is thus made easier, those foods add their energy to the person eating them. Fruits and juices take no more than an hour to digest while vegetables take about 2 hours.

Fresh fruits and vegetables are alkaline-producing foods. They counter the acid-forming foods such as meat, eggs, fish, cheese and game, sugar and flour. Those acid-forming substances are taken to excess by many people, while a raw fruit and vegetable diet acts as an antidote. Natural therapists believe that, in order to keep well, we need a surplus of alkaline-producing foods and that people who follow a conventional diet suffer from an upset of their acid/alkaline balance.

DEAD FOOD

A person feels better eating live foods than after eating a heavy meal consisting of mostly dead foods. Foods that are considered dead are cooked fruits, cooked vegetables and grains, all dairy products, all meat (including fish and chicken), cooked eggs, bread, and soy products (except for edamame). Lightly steamed vegetables are still considered live food. It is recommended to begin weaning oneself away from eating dead foods for better health. Dead foods are mucous-forming in the body as well as acid-producing. This mucous aids in clogging the intestinal system, which can lead to toxicity and other problems.

FRUIT

Fruit needs to be eaten raw, as the body can only utilize fruit in its natural state. Fruit should never be cooked or heat-processed as it becomes toxic and acidic to the body.

SPROUTS

Protein and vitamin levels rise when seeds germinate. In sprouts, then, the level of available proteins and vitamins are very high. Sprouts are an excellent live food, and are already predigested, in other words the body does not need to digest them.

Sprouts help prevent and effect healing against cancer. Two possible reasons for this are chlorophyll and the production of nitriloside in sprouted grains, effective in preventing cancer. Another reason that sprouts may be effective against cancer is that, when sprouts are broken down in the body, they form the chemicals benzaldehyde and cyanide. The normal cells of the body can protect themselves from these chemicals but cancer cells cannot.

Minerals can only be assimilated by the body if they are organic. Eating sprouts lowers the chemical phytin, which prevents absorption of minerals by the body, thus minerals can be more easily assimilated into the body.

Benefits

A diet of live foods can bring relief from osteoarthritis, acute rheumatoid arthritis, chronic rheumatoid arthritis, and muscular rheumatism. Eating live foods brings more energy, clearer thinking, a fresher, more youthful look, and a feeling of lightness.

The world's exclusive and expensive health resorts have known that live foods improve the quality of a woman's life. Two weeks on a raw diet makes a woman look ten years younger— flesh is firmer, lines are softer, and skin, eyes, and hair glow with health. Two years on a high-raw diet can completely transform the shape, texture, and functioning of a woman's body. Cellulite, pre-menstrual tension, hot flashes due to menopause, and excessive menstrual flow can be eliminated without pills or plastic surgery.

Raw energy from live foods can help prevent colds and flu, fight disease, and retard aging. Raw energy can help you shed pounds. It can help banish stress and fatigue, make you feel fitter and younger, and give you a sense of vitality you probably thought you'd never have.

Live foods are extremely cleansing, healthier, and more nutritious. It is suggested that you gradually move to a diet consisting of 70-90 live foods.

Are you a junk food junkie?

You may find it difficult to make the change from cooked, dead food to raw, living food. Dr. Ann Wigmore, a recognized authority on wheatgrass juice and live foods, suggests using a transitional diet which consists of:

- cutting out sugar, milk products, white bread, bakery products, carbonated drinks, hamburgers, hot dogs, alcohol, cigarettes, sugary snacks, canned food, salt, spices, vinegar, coffee and ice cream
- combining food properly
- substituting soups and drinks made from fruit and seeds, wheat or coconut milk; making bread from sprouts; and making candy from dried fruit, fresh coconut, and sunflower seeds
- gradually eliminating meat

- eating celery, vegetables and fruit for snacks when hungry
- fasting for breakfast; then fasting on fruit or water one day a week (see fasting)

MAGNESIUM AND MAGNESIUM SPRAY

If you answer yes to any of the following questions, you may be at risk for low magnesium intake. Do you drink carbonated beverages on a regular basis? Do you regularly eat pastries, cakes, desserts, candies, or other sweet foods? Do you experience a lot of stress in your life, or have you recently had a major medical procedure such as surgery? Do you drink coffee, tea, or other caffeinated drinks daily? Do you take a diuretic, heart medication, asthma medication, birth control pills, or estrogen replacement therapy? Do you drink more than seven alcoholic beverages per week? Older adults are particularly vulnerable to low magnesium status.

Do you experience any of the following?
- Anxiety
- Times of hyperactivity
- Difficulty getting to sleep
- Difficulty staying asleep
- Painful muscle spasms
- Muscle cramping
- Fibromyalgia
- Facial tics
- Eye twitches, or involuntary eye movements

Magnesium oil spray is helpful for those ailments and is:
- Closest to ionic form and easily assimilated by the body
- Tolerated well by those who require large doses of magnesium due to existing deficiencies
- Delivered through the skin and directly available to muscular systems that require magnesium to function

RIFE MACHINE

Dr. Royal Rife invited the Rife machine, which has helped thousands of people around the world recover from serious diseases using his Rife Frequency device. Rife documented a Mortal Oscillatory Rate which would be able to destroy various pathogenic organisms by vibrating them at a particular rate. Rife claimed he could devitalize disease organisms in living tissue.

P.S. I have two dear friends who both have Lyme disease and assert their Rife machines are extremely helpful in controlling this devastating illness.

SERRAPEPTASE

Serrapeptase is a naturally occurring proteolytic enzyme isolated from the digestive system of the silkworm. As a supplement it is used as part of a healthy daily diet and lifestyle, and works by breaking down certain proteins by hydrolysis. The effect of negative protein hydrolysis means you may support normal body processes such as the natural healing process, sinus activity, fluid balance, joint mobility, post-surgical recovery, and anti-inflammation without side effects, waste, and toxin removal. Serrapeptase may help to support and maintain muscle and joint health and promote normal cardiovascular arterial health.

Studies suggest that this enzyme produces anti-inflammatory mediators which reduce swelling, redness, and pain. Serrapeptase contributes to blocking pain-inducing amines from inflamed tissue. People with joint problems and slow healing from injury or post-operative recovery may benefit from nutritional levels of Serrapeptase. Taking this enzyme on an empty stomach is recommended.

P.S. For 15 years I had extreme pain in my chest (costal chondritis) as well as my upper back without much relief. I took pain pills and anti-inflammatories almost daily and went to a physical therapist for days every month. Then I started taking 160,000 IU of serrapeptase daily. Within three weeks the pain was completely gone. I have been symptom-free for 31 months (as of this writing).

SOY PRODUCTS—TOFU, TEMPEH, MISO, TAMARI, EDAMAME

Most vegetables and fruits are not complete proteins and thus cannot be utilized as whole proteins in the body. In vegetarian diets, soy products provide a complete protein to supplement a diet lacking in animal protein. Soy is a vegetable-based protein, combines well with other foods, is easy to use and cook with, and is quite tasty and adaptable. Fermented soy products are also easier to digest than are animal products. Non-GMO soy products are recommended.

Meat eaters who are wanting to cut down on meat consumption or eliminate meat altogether can use soybean products as a substitute vegetable protein source. Macrobiotics uses soy products extensively.

In terms of feeding the world, soybeans are more economical than meat. It is ecologically more efficient to grow soybeans and use its products than it is to raise cattle. An acre of soybeans will feed more people and provide more protein than an acre of land used to feed animals.

Tofu is curdled soybean milk, or soybean curd, cooked to the consistency of hard cottage cheese and almost without flavor. Tofu is extremely versatile. It easily picks up the flavor of herbs and spices that are added to it. It can be cooked, added to casseroles, made into sandwich spreads, and scrambled like eggs. It can be used like meat, in sauces, dressings, and made into mayonnaise. It can be added to soup, salads, eggs, waffles, pancakes, and French toast. Tofu makes delicious desserts, such as cheesecake.

Tempeh is made from inoculating cooked, hulled soybeans with a beneficial mold that binds the beans into a solid compact cake. It has fiber and is a more complete food than tofu. Tempeh is high in B vitamins and protein. Tempeh can be used as sautéed steaks and with other foods.

Miso is a puree made from fermented soybeans and salt. It has a very high ratio of protein to calories and contains high quality protein. Miso is packed full of high energy carbohydrates, few fats, and is unsaturated. It is a well-balanced food. Miso is a delicious, inexpensive, and convenient base for recipes. Its dark or clear broth is rich in minerals and vitamins and makes a delicious soup stock. Miso can be used as a dressing or for seasoning.

Tamari, also known as shoyu or soy sauce, is the liquid which accumulates in miso kegs during the fermentation process. It is used in soups, salads, dressings, used to marinate tofu, sauté, baste, or stir fry, or tamari can be used like a condiment; the list is endless. Tamari has more nutrients in it than the traditional soy sauce sold in grocery stores.

Dashi is a clear soup stock made out of miso and the sea vegetable kombu.

Soy milk is used to replace cow's milk for infants, children, and adults who have allergies to or cannot digest cow's milk. Different flavors such as strawberry, vanilla, and carob have been added to make soy milk a treat. Soy ice cream is available in health food stores and grocery stores.

SPIRULINA; CHLORELLA; MARINE ALGAE

Spirulina is a food, and is found as a blue-green algae that grows in alkaline waters. It is a photo-synthetic organism capable of converting light directly into life and is grown in special ponds. This food comes in a powder form which can be mixed with juices, used in soups and in cooking. It can also be taken in tablet or capsule form.

Spirulina is a highly concentrated source of all vitamins, minerals, digestive enzymes, trace elements, cell salts, and chlorophyll that the body needs for perfect nutrition. The claim is that one could live on 2-3 teaspoons of spirulina per day.

Spirulina is high in beta carotene, which has been found to be effective in protecting against cancer. It is rich in chlorophyll, which is vital for the body's rapid assimilation of amino acids and for the synthesis of enzymes. Spirulina is highly digestible and low in calories, fats, and sodium, and high in efficient protein.

Spirulina contains 18 of the 22 amino acids necessary to construct and maintain the cells of the body, including the 9 essential amino acids that the body cannot manufacture for itself. These 9 amino acids represent a complete protein. Soybeans are more productive per gram than raising animals for meat, and spirulina is more useful than soybeans. One tablespoon of spirulina equals 20-25 grams of vegetable protein which equals 80 grams of meat protein. One acre of spirulina ponds produces over 20 times the protein produced by an acre of soybeans.

Spirulina can be used for a variety of purposes:
- Rich vitamin source
- Concentrated food reserve for snacks, quick pick-me-ups, camping, disaster, and famine relief

- Natural low-calorie supplement for weight control
- Fasting and cleansing—spirulina's other properties encourage intestinal cleansing of the body which is important for a healthy metabolism
- Athletes and bodybuilders can use spirulina for body development and stamina
- Spirulina is beneficial for treating diabetes, anemia, hepatitis, cirrhosis of the liver, pancreatitis, cataracts, glaucoma, ulcers, and gastro ptosis
- Spirulina is healthful for pregnant women and children

Spirulina has been used for centuries in Chad and Ethiopia and is still an important protein source of African people.

It was used by the ancient Aztecs and Mayans. Spirulina has found popularity in Japan, where the Japanese, along with Dr. Christopher Hills in America, have been researching spirulina extensively for the last 38 years. It is being pharmaceutically grown in freshwater ponds in Israel, Taiwan, and the USA.

Deserts could be converted into productive food land by growing spirulina. It is considered by some to be the answer to the planet's hunger and starvation problem, not only because it is easy to grow in the world's deserts, but also because of its nutritional value.

Other types of other blue-green algae are available including chlorella and marine algae.

"The Christopher Hills Foundation has been a non-profit 501(c)3 organization for 38 years, growing and selling Light Force spirulina. Their goal is to carry forward Christopher Hills' vision of a world free from hunger using sustainable technologies to advance humanity. Cyanobacteria cultures developed by Christopher Hills and his partners have benefited millions of hungry refugees, helped people lose weight and even fed astronauts in space."—See more at: http://hillsfoundation.org/#sthash.gK6Gd9tm.dpuf

P.S. A dear friend of mine fed her child a diet of spirulina and juices (rather than milk) from the time he was an infant until about three years old. After he began eating solid foods, he continued to consume a daily spirulina drink. He grew up to be extremely intelligent and has been robustly healthy throughout his life. He is now a computer programmer in Spokane, Washington.

SUPPLEMENTS; VITAMINS; MINERALS

Generally a nutritionist, naturopath, chiropractor, ortho-molecular physician, or preventive medical doctor will prescribe vitamins, minerals, amino acids, glandulars, or other forms of nutritional supplementation. These are found in the form of capsules, tablets, and powder. Paavo Airola, a leading nutritionist, said that because of the poor quality of food, food growing methods, food storage, and preparation today, it is difficult to get all the nutrients one needs solely from food.

When buying any prescribed supplements, it is important to be aware of the following:

1. Although Health Food Stores are excellent places to buy nutritional supplements, you must be sure to READ ALL LABELS. Check to see if there are any substances added to the product that you wish to avoid such as different forms of sugar including fruit and corn sugars (fructose, dextrose and sucrose are some of the names); starches and fillers; yeast; animal products; and food colorings and flavorings. MSG is commonly called "natural food flavoring" and is ubiquitous in many products, while high fructose corn syrup is an additive to most packaged products and is highly toxic.

2. Look at the DOSAGE. If you are supposed to take 50 milligrams of a particular vitamin, for example, check the label to make sure each tablet or capsule contains 50 mg. Sometimes you may find you have to take 2-3 tablets to get the 50 mg. Vitamins that look like a bargain at first glance may actually cost more if you have to double or triple the amount of tablets you take. If B-complex is prescribed, be aware that some brands may have very low dosages of the individual B vitamins. Make sure that the B-complex you are about to buy has dosages that have been prescribed for you, rather than picking up a bottle of B-Complex without checking the label. When you are purchasing a multi-vitamin, check the label. With many brands the dosages are low; double-check with your health practitioner on amount of dosages required.

3. Most of the vitamins on the market are chemically-based. In other words, they are not derived from food but are made in a laboratory. Some people can utilize synthetic vitamins; some cannot. Simply because the vitamin bottle label reads "natural" does not necessarily mean it is made from food products. Many of the vitamins sold in grocery stores and drug stores are synthetic. In order to know if a vitamin is derived from food, you have to READ THE LABEL and know what the name on the label means. For example, Vitamin B-6 is called Pyridoxine Hydrochloride if it is chemically made. Vitamin C that is made from rose hips or acerola cherries is a food-sourced vitamin.

    Vitamins that are manufactured from natural food sources are generally more expensive than the ones that are chemically derived, but the difference in cost seems to be worth it. Their dosages are also lower, but because they are food-derived, their potency and absorption seems to be higher.

4. There has been much research done on Vitamin C. Bioflavonoids, rutin, and hesperidin are substances which are important for the proper assimilation of Vitamin C. Check the label to see if those have been included in your container of Vitamin C. Ascorbic acid, which is one form of Vitamin C, can be irritating to your stomach lining if taken in large dosages. Sodium- , potassium- , calcium- , magnesium- , zinc- , and manganese ascorbates may be substituted for ascorbic acid. Two-time Nobel-prize winner Dr. Linus Pauling studied the effects of Vitamin C, which cannot be manufactured within the human body, but must be supplemented. He recommended a person take at least 4 grams (4,000 mg) of vitamin C per day for optimal health, more to fight cancer and other illness.

5. Talk to your alternative health care doctor or nutritionist regarding the various vitamin combinations that he/she wants you to take. Some vitamins must be combined with other vitamins or minerals in order for the body to make use of them. For example, Vitamin D must accompany calcium in order for the calcium to be absorbed. Yet taking large quantities of calcium depletes the body of magnesium, so must be balanced with magnesium.

6. Some experts feel that B vitamins must be combined (B-Complex) for the full effect of the B-vitamin therapy, rather than taking separate B vitamins such as B-1 or B-12 by itself.

7. B-complex vitamins made from food are far superior to those created in a laboratory. Some theorize that B-complex cannot be absorbed at all unless it is food-based. B vitamins are essential for the health of the central nervous system.

8. Many minerals cannot be absorbed into the body unless they are chelated. Some experts believe that the body cannot absorb minerals that are derived from inanimate sources, such as calcium from oyster shells or dolomite.

9. The minimum daily requirement of vitamins is simply a guide to prevent disease like scurvy and rickets. Your body may require more than the MDR, especially if you are ill.

10. Your doctor or clinic may want to sell their own supplements. That is a good place to start. Keep your wits about you, though.

WATER MACHINES

H2O is the most important nutrient for the body, yet it is the most overlooked. Systems have been designed to incorporate cutting-edge technology to take advantage of the health benefits of making ionized drinking water at home. These machines are simple to install and will provide reliable performance for many years to come. Ionized drinking water offers weight loss and body detoxification, relief from joint pain, and faster re-hydration. Some health-oriented grocery stores are now offering ionized drinking water for sale.

P.S. Kangen water machines are manufactured in Japan, where they are considered a medical device. I'm told every Japanese hospital has Kangen water machines for their patients. The machine alkalizes, ionizes, and oxygenates drinking water. For the last 5 years my own Kangen water machine has helped my health immeasurably and it tastes delicious. I invite you to do your own research on this topic.

WHEATGRASS JUICE

Wheatgrass juice is the sweet, green juice pressed from young wheat plants.

Chlorophyll, a precious folk medicine remedy for many years, is abundant in the green juice of grasses, especially wheatgrass.

Wheatgrass is juiced at the peak of its nutritional value, and it is rapidly assimilated by the body. It is best taken on an empty stomach. There are special wheatgrass juicers on the market, or the fresh grass can be chewed until thoroughly masticated, then spit out. Wheatgrass juice can be purchased in some health food stores, and is also very easy and inexpensive to grow at home. It takes a handful of wheat berries, water, a tray of topsoil, and a cover. Wheatgrass grows in seven days and costs about ten cents a tray. One tray yields about 7–10 ounces of juice. A recommended daily amount of wheatgrass juice is between 1–4 ounces.

Fasting can be done with wheatgrass juice. The cleansing is very thorough and may be accompanied by symptoms which indicate that toxins are being removed. If symptoms show up, do not be alarmed. Get plenty of rest. Drink warm water. Enemas speed up removal of toxins; get massaged; take sponge baths; do body rubs and soak feet. Dr. Ann Wigmore advised her patients to take colonics before starting a wheatgrass juice fast.

Drinking wheatgrass juice will improve sleep and decrease the hours needed for sleep. Wheatgrass juice helps to detoxify the blood and strengthen health. Waste and debris is removed from the body. Wheatgrass juice attacks and destroys bacteria and malignant cells; bolsters the immune system; guards against environmental hazards; builds blood and stimulates circulation; detoxifies the liver; deodorizes body; rejuvenates and extends life; repairs DNA; neutralizes and reverses the accumulation of free radicals in the body.

A scalp treatment can be done with the juice and it can be dropped into the nostrils to clear the sinuses. A few ounces of wheatgrass juice in bath water or rubbed into the skin improves circulation.

Wheatgrass juice is good for bed-ridden patients, people who have lost their appetite, and incurables. Wheatgrass juice benefits people with chronic fatigue, sinusitis, ulcers, and cancer.

INTUITIVE, PSYCHIC, AND SPIRITUAL PRACTICES

There seems to be a whole universe many are not aware of—the world beyond the five senses. I have lived in both the physical "real" world and this hidden world since I was five years old. I believed certain things before I knew there were words for those beliefs. I knew things and saw things I had no way of explaining but which turned out to be accurate. Starting when I was nine my Aunt Edna began to loan me books so I could understand what I was experiencing. Consequently, the arena of extra-senses influenced me, I learned from it constantly, and I gained healing in that area.

People like me are not unusual as we are all intuitive and psychic to some degree. Each of us has five senses and receive input constantly from our environment through those senses.

Some simply have more of a talent for it than others and are extremely sensitive. Input travels through their mind's computer and the information is digested, assimilated, and understood very quickly. Thus, they appear to be psychic. If other people were able to be responsive to the same input and to process as quickly, they would probably come up with the same conclusions as a psychic person.

We each have an indefinable essence in our makeup. I call that spirit. It is who we are beyond our personality and our body. This spirit-self must be in balance with the other levels—physical, mental, and emotional. It also must be nurtured in order for us to be whole and well.

Spirit is all-knowing and may be the link to a Higher Power. When I was desperate, I prayed to be free of pain or illness. The prayer was answered. I was led around, from place to place, person to person, always being given answers, discovering books to read, or finding a therapy that would provide relief and I would follow messages to further healing and serenity.

I have included this section so that you may search deep within yourself, to communicate with that spirit if need be with the help of those talented psychic few. Thus, you may find your truth and your own path to wellness, peace, and happiness.

ASTROLOGY

The principle of astrology is based upon a connection existing between life patterns of human beings and the dynamic patterns of relationship existing within the solar system—the planets, sun, and moon. This connection between planets and ourselves, as shown in one's astrological chart, reveals strengths and weaknesses as well as upcoming trends. Astrology is a tool to realize that we are not at the mercy of the stars, unable to control our own fate. Like those who believe in affirmations, positive thinking, and cognitive awareness, modern astrologers believe that our lives are not determined by the planets but are shaped by our own thought patterns. The planets reflect what is going on, like a mirror. The astrology chart can be a map, a blueprint for discovering who we truly are and who we can become when we decide to take charge of all the internal and external energies affecting us. Using astrology consciously, actively, constructively and responsibly, we can both discover ourselves and work in cooperation with universal forces.

Problems in relationships are probably the single-most cause of misery, depression, and upset in life. One of the most valuable and important contributions of astrology is in promoting better understanding between people through the field of horoscopic comparison. Virtually anyone can be better understood—children, parents, employers, employees, lovers, friends, and mates. Insights can include not only the present, but also past problems, and future trends.

Medical astrology can be extremely valuable. The signs of the zodiac represent certain parts of the body. Using medical astrology, the chart can show weaknesses in the body, glands, and organs as well as potential problems. When an astrologer can "read" those influences in the astrological chart, then the client can know where to take corrective action, diet, exercise, and also to correct his thinking. Foremost astrological expert Edward Doane using the astrological chart could correctly diagnose ailments that had eluded conventional approaches.

Astrology is also a discipline of mind, a technique for development of holistic thinking. Astrology is a study of cyclic patterns, to perceive things as wholes rather than unrelated parts. Through Astrology we may become aware of a unity in the Universe and realize that all things are in some way related to everything else. Or as some New Age philosophers state, everything is connected to everything.

Astrology may be used as a tool for self-actualization. The humanistic approach to astrology sees the person as an independent organic whole consisting of an intricate pattern of interrelated and interacting forces. The birth chart then reflects something that person may become or is in the process of becoming.

Today's astrologers find themselves in esteemed company. Pythagoras, Hippocrates, Plato, Aristotle, Roger Bacon, Thomas Aquinas, Dante, Leonardo Da Vinci, Copernicus, Nostradamus, Galileo, Johannes Kepler, Rene Descartes, Sir Isaac Newton, Edmund Halley (Halley's comet), Goethe, and Carl Jung all studied and promoted astrology. Jung constructed an astrological chart for each of his patients and used that information in therapy.

Most of us live life in the fast lane. Individual and national destinies are moving at an accelerated

rate. One of the branches of astrology, predictive charting—interpreting future tendencies—can be useful. Foreknowledge of upcoming trends can be an invaluable aid to the use of latent opportunities and to the intelligent direction of life.

P.S. My daughter Andrea was born with her sun ruled by the sign Taurus. Not only is her sun in that sign, but several other planets as well. This means she is strongly Taurean. Taurus represents the throat area. For the first four years of her life, Andrea suffered sore throats, tonsillitis, and ear infections on a painfully regular basis. Since I had studied astrology, I knew this was a weak area for her due to influences in her chart. When she turned four, I began to encourage her doctor to take more aggressive action than to continuously give her penicillin, which was losing its effectiveness on her. I also felt it was not healthy for her to receive so much antibiotics into her young body. Finally, the doctor agreed with me, her tonsils were removed, and Andrea has had no further problems with her throat since then.

BIORHYTHM

The biorhythm theory is consistent with biology, which holds that all life consists of the discharge and creation of energy in an alternation of positive and negative phases. Day and night, winter and summer, growing and dying, ebb and flow.

Biorhythm explains that each of us is influenced by three internal cycles—physical, emotional, and intellectual—which we follow from birth until death. The three cycles each follow a different time frame:

The physical cycle takes 23 days to complete and affects a broad range of physical factors, including resistance to disease, strength, coordination, speed, physiology, other basic body function,s and the sensation of physical well-being.

The emotional cycle governs creativity, sensitivity, mental health, and mood, perception of the world and of ourselves, taking 28 days to come full circle.

The intellectual cycle which takes 33 days, regulates memory, alertness, receptivity to knowledge, and the logical, analytical functions of the mind.

The weakest, most vulnerable moments are when each cycle crosses the base line from positive to negative or vice-versa. The base line is the day when each cycle goes into the last half of the phase. For example, the base line for the physical cycle would be the 6th day, (from positive to negative) and the 12th day of the cycle, (from negative back to positive). That day of change is called a critical day.

Accidents, catching colds, and suffering physical harm are examples of physically critical days. Fights, depressions, quarrels, and senseless frustration could occur on emotionally critical days. On intellectually critical days, bad judgment, inability to express oneself, and resistance to learning can be present.

Biorhythms are not things that happen to you. A biorhythm chart is a photographic image of our internal selves. Because biorhythms are connected to energy, it is possible to harmonize with that energy by knowing the ebb and flow, the changing tide of cycles within us. A knowledge of one's biorhythmic fields can be regarded as a tool which will enable you to succeed in getting the best out of yourself in many fields.

A COURSE IN MIRACLES

A Course in Miracles is a three-volume work, channeled by two Columbia University psychologists, which teaches love, oneness, forgiveness, and listening to the inner voice. A Course in Miracles was written as a collaborative venture between Helen Schucman, with portions transcribed and edited by William Thetford. The course came into being through psychic transmissions by Schucman. Thetford then typed the psychic information and helped to arrange it in its present form. This process continued for six years.

According to the Course, sickness is seen as an illusion, and healing is a result of perceiving and understanding that illusion for what it is. Thus, all healing begins in the mind, with the Course as a guide to understanding and perceiving clearly the real world.

The Course teaches that there are two distinct worlds:

- **The real world**—the world of knowledge, truth, and the laws of love
- **The unreal world**—the world of perception, time, and change

The Course states that most of us live in the unreal world, seeing our own beliefs, thoughts, and fears projected outward and experienced as real. The goal of A Course in Miracles is to have the student give up the unreal world and enter a world of universal knowledge or love through the process of changing his perception about the world. The student is thus able to be a source of love. The end result is a happier, healthier view of oneself and the world in general.

The workbook consists of 365 lessons, one lesson for each day of the year, a text in philosophy, and a manual for teachers. The course is designed to be self-teaching, emphasizing experience rather than theory. The text presents a foundation for understanding miracles.

The course makes no claim to finality, nor are the workbook lessons intended to bring the student's learning to completion. At the end, the reader is left in the hands of his or her own internal teacher, who will direct all subsequent learning as he/she sees fit.

P.S. I began hearing about A Course in Miracles in 1986. Many diverse types of people were excited and enthusiastic about that course, from spiritual seekers to psychological counselors, from physicians to massage therapists. The Course changed their lives radically from the old way they had been used to thinking and living.

CRYSTAL WORK AND HEALING; CRYSTAL AND GEM ELIXIRS

Crystals are commercially used today in watches, computer chips, and in lasers. They have been found to be excellent conductors and amplifiers of energy.

In the alternative medical field, crystals are being used for other purposes, such as for healing and meditation. Crystals have an ancient tradition of healing and transformation by organically using stones and crystals. American Indians, ancient Egyptians and Greeks, and Indian and Tibetan Buddhists used them, either by holding the stone in one's hand, laying it on a significant part of the body (i.e., over the heart), or putting it in the bathtub while bathing. The stones and crystals supposedly emit vibrations and frequencies that have powerful, potential effects on the whole being and can be used for healing, transforming, balancing, and attuning body, mind, spirit. Sacred sites are often activated or enhanced by crystalline structures.

Crystals can be used to effect a mood, heal a problem or disease, or to facilitate meditation and dreams. Particular crystals and gemstones are beneficial for recovering from certain types of problems and illnesses, similar to the effects of herbs, flower essence remedies, and homeopathic remedies. Smoky quartz is valuable for all types of healing and is predominately used by crystal healers. Each type of crystal is said to give off a different "vibration" that affects the body/ mind/spirit differently from another crystal. For example, rose quartz gives off a soothing, tender, calm emanation, while citrine energizes.

Each crystal apparently vibrates to a different energy level (chakra) of the body. For example, all the green colored crystals (adventurine, tourmaline, and malachite) vibrate to the 4th (heart chakra) energy center. These green crystals would be useful in cases of heart problems, relationship difficulties, or anything connected to the heart, whether physical, mental, or emotional.

Crystals include quartz, amethyst, lapis lazuli, and tourmaline, just to name a few. Gemstones like rubies, emeralds, and sapphires are also considered to be healing crystals.

Crystals can be placed in strategic places around the home, and worn as jewelry. To wear a crystal on the body is reputed to have that vibration present during the entire time of wearing.

Crystal and Gem Elixirs

Crystal elixirs are prepared by placing a crystal or gemstone in distilled water for two hours, then pouring off the liquid into a clean glass container. The elixir is ingested a few drops at a time, a few times a day, until desired results are achieved. The elixirs can also be added to bath water and to massage oil.

MEDITATION

Inside each of us is a powerful source of knowledge, a self-contained system of help, the Inner Source. Getting in touch with the Inner Source can guide us on how to proceed. If we can learn to trust the Inner Source, it will use a wide variety of systematic, often intricate, and beautiful ways to help us. Meditation is one powerful way of getting in touch with and working with this Inner Source.

Meditation can help us in obtaining inner communion as well as in relieving the ailments which result from the stress and strain of daily living. Attention to our self and our worries can cause stress and tension. Refocusing that attention elsewhere can bring peace, relaxation, relieve us of our anxieties, pain, and illness. Relaxation and refreshment is the beginning of what meditation can do for you, improving total health and well-being, and reducing high blood pressure.

Emotions become more balanced and upsets blow over faster and are less intense when meditating regularly. Meditation enhances self-confidence; people find it easier to handle emotional challenges. Meditation trains the mind to dwell on a new level. The forces of the mind and body become balanced. Meditation can also help develop better concentration, improve work and creativity, and can be used for problem-solving. Meditation can expand to include a feeling of being in oneness and harmony with everyone and everything.

Meditation is not an occult phenomenon, exclusive to a few believers. Meditation occurs spontaneously in daily life and is actually an extension of what we tend to do naturally.

Children and infants can become completely absorbed with some object that has stimulated their curiosity. Geniuses like Newton and Einstein could become engrossed into intense states of absorption. Writers, painters, and dancers can totally immerse themselves in their creative flow, so focused are they on their inner self. Meditation is an innate tendency of the human mind and has been in evidence for thousands of years.

Meditation is divided into three types: dharana, which means concentration in the preliminary stage; dhyana, which means stabilized concentration for a certain length of time; and samadhi, which means complete absorption in one thought or object to the exclusion of every other thought and even sense impressions. Meditation has been called the Yoga of concentration.

The typical technique of meditation is to sit in a relaxed posture and concentrate attention inwardly. That attention may include a mantra, a hymn, the name of God, the sound of nature, or anything outside of ourselves. Many different types of practices are available to learn concentration and mantras. Excellent audio tapes are available to encourage an atmosphere of quiet and peacefulness making it simpler to bring your focus inside. It is recommended to shut your eyes when meditating, making it easier to concentrate and shut out external stimulus.

Meditation should be practiced regularly, at a fixed time and place. A standard length of time to practice meditation is between 5–30 minutes per day. Meditation can also be done with eyes open, in a focused stare, and also while walking. Rhythmic breathing can also be employed during meditation.

At first meditation may be difficult. When you sit still, eyes closed, attention focused inward, you may become aware of the chatter inside your own mind and your body wanting to move. Your mind may want to look everywhere but where you want it to. With time and practice, this mental noise will diminish somewhat, the quiet and stillness of your being will begin to make itself known and you will begin to have control over your thoughts. While meditating, you may become hyper-aware of your body. You may notice every little movement.

P.S. Meditating refreshes me, like having a high-energy nap. I experience feeling less fatigued after I have meditated. My body is rested and my mental and emotional levels are rejuvenated as well. A friend of mine used to call it her 100-yard stare before she knew she was meditating. At those times, she would sit quietly in her living room, staring at the wall, immersed in a deep level of thought which was very comforting and restful to her. Another friend of mine said he did his best meditating while driving his car.

NUMEROLOGY

Numerology is a science of symbols, cycles, and vibration. Scientists and technologists are paying increasing attention to the use of vibrations and frequencies. Numerology is governed by certain rules, based upon facts, of the science or vibrations of numbers.

Numerology is a means of understanding cyclical patterns or qualities that relate to ourselves. It is derived from ancient Hindu teaching, as well as other ancient civilizations. Numerology dates back many years before Christ. Pythagoras and Plato used it. Pythagoras founded a school in approximately 600 B.C., and taught relationships between man and the divine laws reflected in the mathematics of numbers. The Egyptians, Greeks, Romans, and Arabians all had systems of arriving at number vibrations which were remarkably accurate. .

Aspects of nature such as snowflakes, growing plant cells, and the movements of astronomical bodies resonate and relate to numbers. Mathematical resonance occurs widely in such things as sacred geometric frequencies and harmonics, cymatics, fractals, and fundamental energy patterns, as well as the Fibonacci sequence seen in sunflowers and the nautilus shell.

Our own vibrations and cyclical patterns are determined by our date of birth as well as the name on our birth certificate. Numerology reveals certain things about ourselves and our lives, talents and abilities, what our limitations are, what we are here to do and how to accomplish that, careers we are best qualified for, lessons to learn, and karmic debts to pay. Each part of the name and birth date have a meaning and are interpreted differently.

Numerology is simple to learn and understand. Each number has a meaning and a lesson to learn. The digits 1–9 are used, as well as the Master Numbers 11, 22, and 33. When figuring the birth date, all the digits are added together.

The digits are added together again and again until one digit is left. Stop if it is a Master Number —11, 22, or 33.

For example, the birth date 1/7/1947 = 29. Then 29 is added together. 2 + 9 = 11. 11 is a Master Number and is not added again.

When figuring the number of a name, each letter represents a number: A = 1, B = 2, etc. and then beginning again with J = 1, and again at S = 1, through the whole alphabet. The name letters are converted to numbers.

Soul Urge—vowels of name at birth; what we've come to do in our lives.
  For example:
  Mary Jones = 19 (1 + 9) = 1   soul vowels   1 = new beginnings

Personality number—consonants of name at birth. Your Personality number often serves as a censoring device, both in terms of what you send out, as well as what you allow to approach. It lists the characteristics you project and indicates how others are most likely to perceive you before getting to know you well, and so by learning about your Personality Number you can get insight of how others view you.

Destiny number—total of consonants of birth name. It symbolizes the opportunities you have at your disposal, reveals your inner goal, the person you aim to be, and the talents, abilities, and shortcomings that were with you when you entered your human body.

Life Path—total of month, day and year; cosmic report card; what we already know.

Reality number—name and birth path added together.

The birth date number is the most important in Numerology because it cannot be changed like a name can be changed.

PARANORMAL HEALING

Although paranormal healing such as spiritual or psychic healing, psychic surgery, and healing through touch and prayer are considered supernatural or beyond the bounds of scientific explanation, they may be subject to natural laws which are as yet unexplained. The benefits of paranormal healing are widely varied—from healing simple illness to healing disabling diseases such as vascular diseases and cancer.

In a very real sense, medicine is now—as it has always been—faith healing. Without the patient's faith in his physician and the treatment, there can be no hope for cure. Surgeons have long known—we have all known—that the will to live, and faith in the healer and the healing, are essential to recovery.

Faith healing and miracles are a natural phenomenon found in different levels of civilization and among all religions. The roots are tribal in origin. Shamans, medicine men, and witch doctors were thought to be able to diagnose and cure through dreams and trances.

During the time of the Old Testament, the Israelites and Greeks were discouraged from practicing healing. Then Jesus Christ taught his disciples to heal. During the Middle Ages, healing was looked upon as the work of the devil and again discouraged. Physicians came to reject healing, especially the occult practices such as astrology, magic, charms, incantations and trances.

However, in the Christian tradition the laying on of hands and healing through prayer is practiced. Healing shrines exist. Lourdes in France, Compostela in Spain, and the Basilica of our Lady of Guadalupe near Mexico City became famous, and people flocked there for miraculous healing. Today we have charismatic healing, Pentecostal healing, the Quakers and Christian Scientists, and all are accepted as religious forms of healing.

PSYCHIC SURGERY

Psychic surgery is widely practiced around the world, but only has a few practitioners in North America and Europe. Most psychic surgeons are from hot or tropical countries (Brazil, Mexico, and the Philippines).

A psychic surgeon may use a knife or other instrument. He cuts into the patient's body, removes contaminated tissue, repairs what needs repairing, and closes the incision. Sometimes the instruments are crude, like rusty knives and scissors. Many of these surgeons are uneducated, poor people with an extraordinary gift. The most famous psychic surgeon was Arigo, a Brazilian, who claimed a team of doctors worked through him. Although he had only a second grade education and spoke only Portuguese, when healing he spoke fluent German. Arigo and other psychic surgeons have been extensively documented.

This amazing method uses no anesthesia; clients are awake and report they feel very relaxed. There is no pain, sometimes a slight discomfort. Bleeding is minimal. Clients do not go into shock or have any other side effect as in traditional surgery. Although no antiseptic precautions are made, the patient suffers no infections, and the incision heals without scarring.

Another method used widely in the Philippines involves no instrument at all. Philippine healers use their hands for surgery. The body appears to open up to the surgeon's fingers, and closes again afterwards, leaving no scar or wound to heal. Philippine healers reportedly reach into a person's body to remove cancerous masses, cysts, lumps, or other abnormalities of the body.

American healers who use the technique of psychic surgery have a modified version, which they sometimes call etheric surgery. They go into a trance, and perform what looks like a surgical operation, going through motions similar to those which a surgeon could be expected to make but performing them above the patient's body. The theory is they are operating on the spirit body. This spirit body is the body which can be photographed with Kirlian photography, and is reported to leave the physical body at the moment of death.

Normally patients who see these psychic healers have suffered from inoperable tumors or serious disorders which orthodox treatment has failed to treat effectively. Paranormal healing has a reputation for miracles, simply because these healers accomplish what could not be accomplished under normal conditions.

That these miracle workers are able to journey outside of traditional medicine, find the source of the problem, and promote healing suggests there is more to health and disease than is understood at the present time.

REIKI

Reiki is a precise, powerful system of healing which is believed to have originated in Tibet thousands of years ago. It was rediscovered by Dr. Mikao Usui and has achieved popularity in the United States as a contemporary stress management tool, and an overall stimulation to health. The Reiki techniques are used for healing of others by therapists, health practitioners, and lay persons. It is a system of healing which is linked to the human energy field. The interest in Reiki comes for a variety of reasons: People feel uplifted by the treatments they have received. Attunement to the energy is a process available to anyone and can never be lost. To activate one's connection requires only that the hands be placed upon another living object including oneself. Simple, effective, consistent and affordable. Reiki is similar to spiritual healing, the laying on of hands.

Reiki is a tool for mental, emotional, spiritual, and physical balance. Effective as a stress management tool, Reiki promotes an increase in energy and wellness levels, and creates harmonious situations and relationships as well. One Reiki technique works especially on emotional, mental, and addictive problems and another is helpful in alleviating pain.

SOUND HEALING; MUSIC THERAPY; NEW AGE MUSIC; CHANTING

Sound influences us in every area of life, whether it is music, a tonal harmony of many sounds, or noise—sound gone crazy in disconnectedness. Sounds of nature, water, birds, and insects impact us in a certain way, just as sounds of traffic, crowds, or pots and pans clashing affect us in a different way. Sound as music can be soothing, healing, or energizing, but noise can also disturb us. Sound therapy or music therapy has beneficial applications that can heal body, mind, and spirit.

From ancient civilizations such as Greece to the Renaissance to modern times, music has evoked sensations, moods, and emotions. Music can increase mood, bring it to climax, or dispel it entirely.

Music has many wonderful and distinctive qualities. It can intensify our feelings, summon to mind associated images and memories, transport us into a state of awe, or simply charm us through the delicacy of melody. In primitive trance rituals, frantic monotonous drumming can lead mediums into a trance state. Researchers believe that pain-killing endorphins may be released when the brain's pleasure center is activated by the aesthetic sensations of music. Some music therapists are so skilled that patients are able to stop taking painkillers.

Helen L. Bonny, founder of the Institute for Consciousness and Music Results, has a music prescription. Her research showed that music helped to reduce heart rate, produced positive effects on depression, anxiety, and the relief of pain. Blood pressure and pulse rates were lowered, breathing became regular and deep, muscles relaxed, and patients were found to sleep better. Nurses found it easier to change IV's when patients were listening to soothing music.

Hospitals are allowed to invite musicians. Doctors at the Kaiser-Permanente Medical Center in Los Angeles, California, prescribe music tapes instead of pain killers and tranquilizers. Playing music during an MRI is encouraged.

NEW AGE MUSIC

Much New Age music is designed for a specific purpose such as:
- guided imagery and visualization

- shamanic healing
- meditative
- basic relaxation and stress reduction
  pain reduction

There are five qualities that music contains and these traits are what affects us:

Pitch—acts on a purely physical level in a rational way.

Intensity—an obliterate unwanted sounds; indicate power and make impression or intimacy, quiet, and serenity.

Interval—pleasant or unpleasant; suggests movement, conflict or resolution; stimulating or irritating.

Duration and Rhythm—easy to observe, diverse. Hysterical behavior or hypnotic calm. Sleep can be induced. A repetitive rhythm can be depressing. A strong rhythm suggests will-power and self-control.

Tone—(timbre—non-rhythmical; sensuous; pleasurable; non-intellectual impression.

Chanting—In India and the Orient, chanting is considered to have a positive advantage on health and peace of mind. A chant combines sounds with words, usually repeated. Chanting is customarily done during meditation or ceremonies. The first approach to meditation requires that the attention be focused on a meditation symbol, like a sound or chant.

A mantra consists of set words forming a chant, and is usually Chinese, Indian or Yogic in tradition, although some Christian songs could be considered mantras. A mantra, which is chanted repetitiously, is of ancient lineage. Repetition of this mantra is a convenient and effective way of establishing the crucial relationship and wakening the inner power of healing. The East Indian mantra OM, used while chanting, is considered powerful because "OM" is thought to be the name of God or the sound of the Universe. Indian mantras are used to focus the mind and lead it through its many distractions to a state of inner peace and unity. The chanter does not need to understand that which he is chanting. The subtle vibrations of mantras are intensified by thoughts on the intention of the chant rather than precise pronunciation and rhythm.

Singing and laughing is thought to clear out the liver and detoxify the body. Norman Cousins incorporated laughing when he worked on healing his cancer.

Toning is making sounds with the voice, but without words, syllables, meanin, or form, and can have a beneficial effect upon the body. Several pyramids in Egypt can reflect toning sounds and make it seem as if there are a number of voices with a number of pitches coming back to you instead of just your own. Flautist Paul Horn recorded songs inside the Great Pyramid which sound like a number of flutes. The Grateful Dead also recorded in Egypt.

P.S. A friend of mine had elective surgery. She decided she didn't want surgery room chatter or negative conversation to interfere with her surgery and her healing afterwards. She talked to her surgeon and asked him if he and his staff would only talk in a positive way while they operated on her, saying things like "I can see that she is going to heal very quickly and painlessly." She also asked if she could bring her CD player into surgery and play some of her soothing New Age music tapes. Her doctor agreed wholeheartedly with all of her requests. Her surgery went flawlessly. She was out of recovery very quickly, left the hospital sooner than expected, and had a minimal amount of pain and discomfort. Her surgical wound healed faster than either she or her doctor expected, and healing was rapid and easy. She has only pleasant feelings about her surgery.

SPIRITUAL and PSYCHIC HEALING

According to spiritual healers, all forms of healing come from God to heal the sick. Healers themselves possess no power to heal. They are simply human instruments, and as such healing is not miraculous; the healing is God's law in operation. It is the transfer of the Universal Life Force energy from the healer to the patient.

The spiritual healer is passive. He need not have any medical training or knowledge. The healing energy passes through the healer and into the sick person's body.

Sometimes a spiritual healer may go into a trance (such as Edgar Cayce), talk in a different voice, even report that there are other beings, angels, or doctors who are assisting in the diagnosis and cure of the problem. Spiritualists believe there is a latent capacity in people which can be aroused by the divine healing force—even in those who are unaware of the force's existence. A state of healing inertia may exist with people who have been ill over a considerable length of time. This inertia can be broken through. The mind and the healing intelligence can be re-aroused, and a flow of healing energy from spirit can be induced. Physicians sometimes call this spontaneous healing.

The sick person can be healed by the hands-on method. Some healers place their hands over the patient's body; others do a gentle form of physiotherapy. Patients may feel a coldness or a warmth emanating from the healer's hands; they may feel energized or very relaxed. Usually healing will involve a few booster treatments to complete the healing and keep the patient from reverting back to illness.

Sometimes a healing may take place over great distances. The energy that is transmitted is similar to a radio wave. Healing by prayer usually involves distance.

A patient can connect with his own healing intelligence and do spiritual healing on himself as well as visiting the healing shrines listed above.

SPIRITUAL and PSYCHIC COUNSELING

Many alternative healers and some doctors are aware that from time to time they can accurately diagnose a patient in a flash of intuition or extrasensory perception (ESP). A psychic can diagnose and prescribe for a patient, usually without benefit of medical training and sometimes even without seeing the patient. This information comes in the form of feeling (clairsentient), words (clairaudient) or pictures (clairvoyant).

The most famous psychic diagnostician was Edgar Cayce, a medically untrained man from Kentucky, who could lay down on his couch, go into trance, and diagnose problems which had baffled physicians, and then offer revolutionary cures. His work was completely documented and his unusual cures are still being used for sick people today. His recorded work is the basis for the Association for Research and Enlightenment in Virginia Beach, Virginia.

Other reasons a person may have a psychic or spiritual reading are for problems other than physical such as emotional distress, relationship, or monetary problems.

There is a theory on how a psychic reading works. The theory is that we are all One. We are each surrounded by an energy field, which is in touch with the energy fields of other people. The healer enters into a rapport with the patient's energy field via his own, and is able to ask about the other's physical, mental, and emotional condition. Since he is united with the patient, he intuits the answer. A medical intuitive is considered such a person.

Psychics sometimes use tools in their diagnostic work. Some of the tools available are pendulums (known as radionics), tarot cards, and handling the personal effects of the patient (jewelry, watch, picture, etc.), known as psychometry.

Research is being conducted on the whole paranormal field in the United States and Russia.

Scientists want to understand why and how paranormal practices works. Someday paranormal diagnosing and medicine may be as widely used and accepted as traditional medicine is today.

TAROT

Tarot is an ancient system of divination with picture cards showing symbolic figures, representing stages of man's destiny, as well as vices, virtues, and elemental forces.

The Tarot is thought to have originated from the Qabalah, ancient Hebrew writings. From this ancient teaching, the Tarot was formulated with two things in mind. First, the symbols of humankind are in picture form and second, the occult meanings of numbers, similar to numerology, were included.

In a Tarot deck, there are 56 cards called the Minor Arcana, which in the Middle Ages were used by royalty and contain royal symbols of Kings, Queens, Knights, and Pages. The Minor Arcana in the Tarot is symbolized by Scepters (or Wands), Cups, Swords, and Coins (or Pentacles) which are called Clubs, Diamonds, Spades ,and Hearts in the playing cards of today. The Minor Arcana also symbolize the four elements: fire, earth, air, and water and is similar in that respect to astrology.

The remaining 22 cards of the Tarot are called the Major Arcana and represent pictorial images and dreams plus numbers. It is a symbolic wheel of the opposites of human life.

The Tarot uses symbols from: 1) the Archetypal world of pure ideas 2) the creative world, where ideas become specialized 3) the formative world in which ideas can be expressed 4) the material world which takes the ideas of the worlds and brings them into physical form.

The Tarot is not intended for fortune-telling. To do so is to debase oneself spiritually. Rather than foretelling the past, present, or future, there is a deeper, more esoteric, philosophical purpose. Using the Tarot could be likened to a form of meditation, to dwell more deeply on the meaning of a card as it comes up in a spread of cards.

Indeed, many of the modern Tarot decks suggest that the person contemplate the meaning of each card in a display to fully understand the message to that individual. To use the Tarot in this way can lead a person to find answers within himself, with a Tarot card being the doorway or messenger, to understand and know about himself. With that in mind then, Tarot can be used as a valuable tool in spiritual and psychic counseling and meditation. The Tarot can be used to uncover problems and habit patterns that may affect all areas of health. It can pinpoint psychological sources of illness and determine which areas of the body need to be balanced.

There are many types of Tarot decks, some standard, dating back hundreds of years, others more recent and modernized. Many of the contemporary decks have new symbolism, up-to-date messages and are cast into readings somewhat differently.

TWELVE-STEP PROGRAMS

Another method of spiritual healing exists, although it's not usually considered as such to the lay person. This is the 12–step programs of Alcoholics Anonymous, Overeaters Anonymous, Gamblers Anonymous, and other anonymous programs, with their associated programs of Al-Anon, O-Anon, etc., for families and friends. These are self-help programs that have been instrumental in aiding countless addicts to recover from their diseases and assisting their friends and families to cope with their own experience with the illness.

12–step programs are spiritual in nature. The first step is when the patient acknowledges he is powerless over his addictions. The second step asks that a Higher Power help in healing the disease, whether that disease is alcoholism, compulsive overeating, or being co-dependent. The other 10 steps are involved in understanding oneself, taking responsibility for problems, making amends, and then working out one's life without the disease. 12–step programs have helped people work miracles in their lives in overcoming disabling addictions. Working the steps is a critical component to those miracles.

EXERCISE, MOVEMENT, AND SPORTS

Traditional as well as non-traditional medicine and health care stress the importance of adequate exercise. Aerobics is a popular way to improve physical health. In addition to aerobics, new types of exercise include forms of dance which are stimulating to health and vitality, while incorporating mental, social, and spiritual activity. Some movements are geared to have low impact on the body, which is healthful. Many of these are fun, as well as healthy, and can be done with a partner or in groups.

Exercise not only stimulates the blood and oxygen supply, it also aids in metabolism, digestion, and elimination functions in the body.

Paavo Airola, a noted nutritionist, stated that it is extremely important to get both proper nutrition and proper exercise. However, he believed that if a person only picked one or the other, it would be better to get proper exercise with poor nutrition, rather than good nutrition with little or no exercise. (No, I am not suggesting you eat a junk-food diet while you run every day.)

A side benefit of the exercise practices in this section is that movement and exercise tend to reduce stress, while inducing peace of mind, relaxation, and calmness.

AEROBICS

In the 1960s there was a dramatic increase in deaths from heart attacks in young men 25–44 years old. A study showed that the conditioned heart seems to function most efficiently at a minimal heart rate between 175 and 190 heartbeats during exercise. Conditioning the heart was assumed to lead to better health and longer life.

The word coined for conditioning the heart was called Aerobics, exercise during which the energy needed by the body is supplied by the oxygen inspired into the lungs. Aerobic exercise over an adequate time period increases heart and lung activity and produces beneficial changes in the body. Running, swimming, cycling, jogging, walking briskly, sports, and energetic gardening are all excellent forms of aerobics.

Aerobics lowers blood pressure, provides more energy, burns off calories, helps in weight loss, and has been found to reduce anxiety in senior citizens better than tranquilizers.

Alternative health educators are discovering that exercise is important for proper body metabolism, aids digestion, and is significant in over-all body health.

For proper aerobic functioning one must:
- rapidly breathe large amounts of air
- forcefully deliver large volumes of blood
- effectively deliver oxygen to all parts of the body

Certain points should be followed in aerobic training:
- progress slowly
- warm up properly
- exercise within one's own tolerance
- cool down slowly
- condition to increasing amounts of exercise
- if over 40 or under a doctor's care, it's recommended to have a doctor's supervision.

The first six weeks on an aerobic program can be the hardest. Aerobic exercise only needs to be practiced every other day to be effective. The resting day allows the body to condition itself which is also valuable to health.

Different forms of aerobic exercise include:

W.E.T. —Water Exercise Techniques is an exercise that is practiced in a pool, thereby providing a natural resistance to help tone and strengthen muscles. The risk of injury is eliminated or lessened. There is no strain, while the water is peaceful to the mind. W.E.T. helps to support and relax muscles, and heals injuries faster.

Dance—Another popular form of aerobic exercise is dancing aerobically to music. Special steps are learned for extra benefit to coordination, memory, grace, and fun. Also, there are step aerobics, sport aerobics, and low impact aerobics.

AIKIDO

Aikido is a combination of methods derived from T'ai Chi Ch'uan, Jiu Jitsu, Kendo (sword fighting), and other mental energy techniques. Aikido uses practical self-defense techniques, and is different from the other techniques in that it is totally defensive. There is no attack in Aikido.

Aikido is a martial art form founded in Japan by Ueshiba Morihei, a teacher and philosopher who died in 1969. Aikido means literally the method of coordinating one's spirit. In Aikido, the spirit rules the body and it is of the utmost importance to unify these two forces.

Aikido is not only an excellent self-defense form, but helps a person gains a new sense of harmony with his surroundings. Because of that philosophy, it has gained much popularity with people interested in exercise, coordination, and body mastery.

In Aikido the opponent's force is used against him to throw him off balance, like judo. It is important to remain centered in Aikido. Using one's energy rather than muscles will prevent strains or injuries. The physical training consists of being able to respond to an attack effectively, free the energy trapped in tense muscles, and feel the flow of breath and energy throughout the body. The exercises build strength, flexibility, and agility, although the goal is to integrate body and mind, and use body and mind in a relaxed, non-tense way.

All moves are in accordance with the laws of nature. When body and spirit are unified, it helps to overcome sickness. As with other movement modalities, like yoga and t'ai chi, Aikido helps to unify the body/mind connection. When that is accomplished, peace of mind and increased health are the result.

EGOSCUE METHOD

The Egoscue Method, developed by Peter Egoscue, has offered non-medical pain relief since 1971. This easy and gentle method has a high success rate without the use of drugs, surgery, or manipulation. The patient is taught how to regain control of his health without becoming dependent on another person or a machine.

The metabolism and immune system as well as every other system in the body are directly linked to posture. The Egoscue Method is basically a set of prescribed stretches utilizing gravity that puts one's body back into a natural alignment and function of posture. Rather than using manipulation, massage, or any other technique, Egoscue strengthens the appropriate muscles which then can be used to pull the body back into alignment.

The body has an amazing ability to heal itself. The body is made to move and, according to Egoscue, there are zero design flaws. The Egoscue method's approach is to eliminate pain while striving to return the patient to as close to that flawless design as possible. Egoscue helps athletes return to competition pain-free while decreasing their chances of future injury by using the Egoscue Method to enhance performance and extend their career.

For someone who wants to increase energy level and improve overall health, Egoscue helps to tap into the body's ability to not only rid itself of pain, but also heal itself of disease and sickness.

INVERSION THERAPY/GRAVITY GUIDANCE

Because of the flexibility of the human body, we can achieve an unlimited number of postures within the full range of gravitational possibilities. Inversion Therapy believes that people can equalize body stress by changing body position and using the force of gravity in a positive way.

There are two sets of postures. First is the common postures, which are comprised of sitting, standing, lying down, and bending forward.

The second set is called the uncommon postures and they are used for countering the effects of gravity. This includes bending backwards, hanging by either set of limbs, standing on hands, forearms, or hanging by the lower limbs. These uncommon postures are to be done daily to maintain health. With both the common and uncommon postures, there is a similarity between this type of movement and yoga.

The gravity guidance system of exercise is the result of 28 years of research by R. Manatt Martin, M.D., D.O., D.C. Dr. Martin's methods of physical fitness enable individuals to not only live more harmoniously with the effects of gravity, but to actually utilize gravity as a tool working for their benefit. After being faced with numerous cases of back pain, Dr. Martin began to draw on his past experience as a gymnast to devise a system of exercise which would help alleviate the downward pull and accompanying pain of the force of gravity. Dr. Martin has invented exercise equipment to help people. Inversion boots, also known as anti-gravity boots, and inversion swings are two of these.

This method may be an alternative to back braces and surgery, and can help prevent back problems, and maintain good muscle tone and conditioning. Before beginning inversion therapy, consult with a health practitioner.

QIGONG

Qigong is an ancient Chinese health care system that integrates physical postures, breathing techniques, and focused intention. The word Qigong is made up of two Chinese words. Qi is pronounced chee and is usually translated to mean the life force or vital-energy that flows through all things in the universe. The second word, Gong, pronounced gung, means accomplishment or skill that is cultivated through steady practice. Together, Qigong means cultivating energy. It is a system practiced for health maintenance, healing, and increasing vitality.

Qigong is an integration of physical postures, breathing techniques, and focused intentions. The various Qigong practices can be classified as martial arts, medical, or spiritual. All styles have three things in common: they all involve a posture, (whether moving or stationary), breathing techniques, and mental focus. Some practices increase the Qi, others circulate it, use it to cleanse and heal the body, store it, or emit Qi to help heal others. Practices vary from the soft internal styles such as T'ai Chi; to the external, vigorous styles such as Kung Fu. However, the slow gentle movements of most Qigong forms can be easily adapted, even for the physically challenged and can be practiced by all age groups.

Qigong creates an awareness of and influences dimensions of our being that are not part of traditional exercise programs. Most other forms of exercise do not involve the meridian system used in acupuncture nor do they emphasize the importance of adding mindful intent and breathing techniques to physical movements. When these dimensions are added, the benefits of exercise increase exponentially. The gentle, rhythmic movements of Qigong reduce stress, build stamina, increase vitality, and enhance the immune system. It has also been found to improve cardiovascular, respiratory, circulatory, lymphatic, and digestive functions.

T'AI CHI

Developed in China centuries ago, T'ai Chi is a system of exercise that makes use of the entire body. Movement is very slow and deliberate, continues without break or pause, and the person uses concentration and awareness while performing. The movements are circular and gentle, done in an even, slow tempo synchronized with your breathing. T'ai Chi is done almost leisurely without any special muscular effort. The movements ensure that the person remains balanced.

T'ai Chi increases body/mind coordination so that energy can be more efficiently utilized. This leads to peacefulness and better health. The body moves as a unit and vitality is increased. Muscle tone is increased and circulation is improved. It opens up the joints and alleviates joint disease, especially in the knees, and straightens the spine.

Since this exercise causes no strain, T'ai Chi is prescribed for heart disease, palpitations, angina, and hypertension. It is an excellent alternative to tranquilizers.

T'ai Chi stimulates the nervous system and increases the blood circulation and glandular activity. It strengthens muscles, exercises the joints, and retards the aging process. It eases tension, calms the heart, and coordinates the mind and body.

There are two main forms used in the West today. One is T'ai Chi Ch'uan, developed by Yang Lu-Ch'an, during the Chou Dynasty (1066-403 B.C.). This is a series of specific ritualized patterns of flowing movement called forms. The long form of Tai Chi Chiuan consists of 108 movements.

The short form is 37 movements which can be completed in 7–10 minutes.

The other type of T'ai Chi popular today is T'ai Chi Chih. This uses all the major movements of T'ai Chi Ch'uan, but there is no set pattern to the movements and they are done at random.

T'ai Chi has been called "meditation in motion." Its movements are similar to Kung Fu and dance therapy and use both meditation and martial arts techniques. The secret of T'ai Chi is tranquility. All movements should be performed with a relaxed mind and body. Maximum effect comes from minimum effort.

T'ai Chi can be practiced anywhere, indoors or out. 15–20 minutes daily is all that is needed. Loose fitting clothing is recommended. All ages can practice T'ai Chi and gain the benefits.

YOGA

The yoga tradition maintains that there is a mechanism in each of us which brings balance to the body and mind and integrates the functioning of the two. Every person has this power to adapt, no matter what the stimulus, circumstances, or irritation that is present in life. The body and mind attempts to restore balance no matter what is happening internally or externally.

Yoga is a way to assist the body and mind to maintain their state of balance, or if lost, regain it quickly, regardless of any disturbing factors present in the person's life. Yoga helps with weight loss, firms muscle tone, promotes healthy skin, good posture, flexibility, grace, poise, coordination, voice, vitality, and promotes better sleep. Yoga can help to detoxify the body. Pregnant women can benefit from yoga. All ages can enjoy yoga.

On a non-physical level, yoga enables a person to deal with problems better, to relax, relieve physical stress, increase creativity, and relieve emotional stress and specific tensions.

Yoga is a physical, mental, and spiritual experience all at the same time. It is easily incorporated into one's lifestyle. The exercises and postures, called asanas, are based on natural movements of the body and involve stretching. The asanas teach control, concentration, and mastery of the body. Yoga exercises the inner organs as well as the outer body. Yoga includes breathing techniques, mental focus and concentration, and meditation.

The different types of yoga are:

- hatha yoga (most common)—asanas and breathing, body control
- mantra yoga—repetition of sounds and mystical phrases
- laya yoga—inward, imaginary sound
- shiva yoga—inward concentration
- bhakti yoga—spiritual perfecting in daily life
- karma yoga—service to others
- raja yoga—mental control
- kundalini yoga—arousing the latent internal power to produce illumination through breathing and concentration on the nerve plexuses in the spine and head

The tradition of yoga began in Northern India over 5,000 years ago. Philosophers, scholars, and warriors who examined the ephemeral quality of life, with its inevitable sufferings and tragedies, sought to give it deeper meaning and purpose. Indian philosopher Patanjali formulated yoga into a science during the 2nd century BCE.

P.S. Yoga helps with back problems. My work supervisor attended yoga classes regularly. She became acquainted with a man at her class. He had been practicing yoga for years and was quite limber. When she got to know him better, he told her that he had severe back problems and had been in pain a good deal. His doctor had recommended yoga to him. Within a short while, his back loosened up, the pain dissipated, and he's been practicing yoga ever since. His elderly parents attended yoga classes with him.

NATURAL CHILDBIRTH

Natural childbirth has expanded over the last few decades. It is childbirth without pain and/or without needing drugs or anesthesia. Childbirth coaching may be included and is often provided by the baby's father, someone close to the family, or a professional labor coach.

In recent years there has been a growing desire among prospective parents to give birth in an intimate setting with family members. Consequently, there has been an upsurge in home births and in comfortable, homey birthing centers, where relatives, friends and other children of the new parents can watch and even participate in the birth experience.

Birthing chairs permit the mother to sit upright, which improves efficiency and the comfort of the mother during labor.

Yoga, T'ai Chi, and the Alexander technique can be helpful for the mother to learn relaxation and calmness, to practice non-stressful exercise, and to stretch the muscles prior to delivery, all for more ease during childbirth.

Conscious breathing (rebirthing) has found a niche in natural childbirth for two reasons. The first is that the mother can release her own birth trauma prior to delivery, allowing her to more fully and consciously be supportive of herself and her baby. The second is that the breathing techniques used in conscious breathing aid in relaxation and pain reduction. Both the Bradley and LaMaze methods use conscious breathing as a tool.

Massage, during labor and after childbirth as well as for pre-natal care, is practiced in births of newly developing countries. The benefits of this type of massage are being incorporated here in the United States for healthier mothers and babies. Infant massage is being promoted to decrease birth trauma and to develop bonding between child and parents.

UNDERWATER BIRTHING

A water birth means at least part of a mother's labor, delivery, or both happen while she's in a birth pool filled with warm water. The birth can take place in a hospital, a birthing center, or at home. A doctor, nurse-midwife, or midwife helps the mother through the delivery.

In the U.S., some birthing centers and hospitals offer water births. Birthing centers are medical facilities that offer a more homelike setting than a hospital and more natural options for women having babies.

The use of a birthing pool can:
• Help ease pain
• Keep a mother from needing anesthesia
• Speed up labor

Any of the natural childbirth methods and techniques above can be combined. Only the preference of the parents can decide which methods they want to utilize. A relaxed, humane, happy, painless, loving, and safe environment for both mother and child is the focus of natural childbirth.

BRADLEY METHOD

Dr. Robert Bradley uses similar methods as La Maze. He encourages natural healing afterwards, and he emphasizes the joy of having a baby, rather than focusing on fear, pain, and the dependency on drugs. The aim is to enable pregnancy and birth to proceed with a minimum of interference. Help is given to prepare a mother in understanding the bodily changes and emotional experiences of pregnancy and to become aware of her responsibility to herself and the developing baby and to be an active participant rather than a patient, so that the birth experience is one of total fulfillment for mother and child.

LA MAZE METHOD

Dr. LaMaze, founder of the LaMaze method of natural childbirth, includes breathing techniques and exercises to strengthen abdominal and perineum muscles to aid in birth process and recovery afterwards. LaMaze teaches relaxation methods and ways for the labor coach to help the mother be more comfortable during labor and delivery. LaMaze stresses the importance of knowledge— being aware of different body changes and the various stages of labor preceding birth, and encourages knowing what to expect during pre-natal and post-natal periods as well.

LEBOYER METHOD

Dr. LeBoyer emphasizes sensitivity not only to the mother, but to the baby as well. The newborn baby is not at all the unconscious thing we have assumed it to be. We have assumed that a newborn baby doesn't feel, see, hear, and has no emotions. It is just the opposite. A baby still has a consciousness which is wide open, not conditioned or protected, and this is what can make birth traumatic. The senses of the newborn baby are so open, sensitive, and sharp that all stimuli must be kept as minimal as possible.

Using the LeBoyer method, lights are dimmed in the delivery area. Noise is kept to a minimum. Talking is low and calm. The staff proceed peacefully. When the child is born, the umbilical cord is left intact. The child is connected to its mother's breathing until it can breathe on its own. The child is gently touched and talked to by parents and the medical team. This method is aimed at making the birth transition easier and painless for the child, and more humane for all involved.

The umbilical cord is cut after it stops pulsing, usually 5–10 minutes after birth. This alleviates the panic or anguish of the child having to breathe on its own too quickly. The child, which had been lying on its mother's stomach, is picked up gently by the father, and cradled in a warm tub of water. The baby learns to bond with its father and to gain trust and acceptance of the outside world in a pleasurable way. After a few minutes, the baby begins to look around, eyes open (unlike normal pictures of newborns), and even begins to splash and play in the water. The face is calm and happy. Many times, the baby does not even cry during and after birth.

With the LeBoyer method, bonding is stressed as important, both between mother and child, as well as between father and child. The goal is to keep the birth trauma, believed to be the single-most cause of emotional and psychological problems, at a minimum. It may be possible to alleviate many of one's problems before they begin.

MIDWIFERY

Since time immemorial midwives have been around at birthing time. A woman who had particular interest or attunement emerged as the local midwife. Sometimes a woman became a midwife out of a desire to establish a rapport system for mothers-to-be. Sometimes a mother awakens, through her own birthing experience, to a desire to share and facilitate.

The midwife gives thorough pre-natal care, becoming familiar with the couple and any possible complications, as well as providing birth and post-partum care. The advocates of midwifery offer that midwives are women with their own experience of birthing and, as such, are more supportive, understanding, and empathetic to the mother than male doctors.

Because of an upsurge in midwifery, there may not be a doctor in attendance. Sometimes the doctor will only be present at the birth itself, not during pre-natal, labor, or post-natal periods. Sometimes birth attendants are nurse-midwives with a doctor in attendance. The method and mode of learning to be a midwife is highly individual, usually beginning as an apprentice to another midwife. The apprentice must learn to deal with complications, provide care for the infant, and repair tears in the vaginal wall.

PRIMAL THERAPY

Primal therapy as created by Dr. Arthur Janov examines the power of beliefs and how they are used as a mechanism for dealing with early trauma that goes as far back as birth and even into the womb, and reveals that love is a biological need.

Life before Birth, authored by Dr. Janov, explains in detail how early trauma and adversity can have lifelong consequences and result in serious afflictions from cancer to diabetes. Events during pregnancy may be as important, if not more important, than genes in determining mental illness, heart, respiratory problems, diabetes, Alzheimer's and even the length of one's life.

NON·INVASIVE TESTING

In terms of health, non-invasive testing does not invade the body or have potentially dangerous side effects, as do X-rays, MRI's, CAT scans, angiograms, exploratory surgery, etc.

Non-invasive health tests are valuable in determining health problems but pose little or no threat to one's well-being. For example, x-rays invade the body and can be dangerous, particularly if a patient is pregnant or if a person is exposed to too many x-rays. On the other hand, thermography is a non-invasive test. It does not harm or invade the body at all; it merely records the heat emissions of the various parts of the body to determine problems like loss of circulation or hardening of the arteries.

Non-invasive testing can be subtle and can ascertain health problems that traditional invasive testing cannot. With sensitive testing available today, many diseases can be detected in their earliest stages, long before they produce disabling diseases. In some cases, non-invasive health tests may be able to replace traditional health tests.

Non-invasive testing is relatively painless and not unpleasant. Some non-invasive testing techniques are:

APPLIED KINESIOLOGY/MUSCLE TESTING

When doctors use traditional testing methods, they cannot always determine the exact causes of their patients' symptoms. Applied kinesiology differs from other tests because it provides a means of obtaining a response from the body itself.

Applied kinesiology works for both diagnosis and treatment of weaknesses and imbalances. New treatment systems that were once only theoretical developed out of this testing technique. Allergies, particularly food allergies, are now easily detected and greatly helped through applied kinesiology. Nutritional deficiencies can be determined through muscle testing. Misalignments of the skeleton, deficiencies of hormones and enzymes, uneven muscle development, and destructive thought patterns can be found. Muscle testing can enable practitioners to detect malfunctions of the body long before they become acute enough to cause actual clinical symptoms such as pain or weakness.

Applied kinesiology is a method of investigating body function which uses the muscles of the body to test the body's different nerve and energy patterns. When a nerve or energy pattern is functioning improperly, the muscle being tested appears weak. When the appropriate test is used or correction is made, the muscle becomes amazingly strong in comparison to its previous status. The reverse is true when a nerve or energy pattern is not adequate to meet the body's demands. A challenge to that energy pattern makes a previously strong muscle become temporarily weak. This system provides the doctor with knowledge in the kinesiology procedures with the ability to locate improper body function and, most of the time, return it to its normal functioning. Muscles are systematically tested and weaknesses are identified and treated, thereby correcting imbalances in the body's energy systems.

Dr. George Goodheart, a chiropractor from Michigan, accidentally discovered the principles of applied kinesiology. He discovered that some of the standard muscle tests he used provided clues to the workings of the entire body. Goodheart began to teach his new findings to other chiropractors. One of them, Brian Butler, introduced Touch for Health in Britain as a result of applied kinesiology techniques. Prior to Dr. Goodheart's findings, it was assumed that backaches and associated problems were a result of muscle spasm or tautness of the muscles. Dr. Goodheart found that the cause was weak muscles on the opposite side of the body, which caused the normal muscles to seem to be, or to become, tight.

A machine, invented and researched in Europe, is available here in the U.S. It is called a hololinguistic processor (trade name Interro) and is connected to a computer and printer. Using the same meridians that muscle testing utilizes, the Interro tests electrical impulses on the meridians to determine deficiencies in nutrition as well as toxicity and allergies. It also then can prescribe what methods could cure these problems and deficiencies. Although the machine is being used for diagnosis by chiropractors, medical doctors and dentists are the only practitioners who can prescribe drugs and treatment using it.

CYTOTOXIC FOOD ALLERGY TESTING

Cytotoxic testing is done with a sample of blood to determine levels of sensitivities and allergies to various foods. The test can be done quickly in the laboratory using only one blood sample from each patient, to avoid possible allergic reactions. A drop of blood is then exposed to various food extracts. By observing the reaction of the patient's white blood cells to different food extracts, hundreds of foods can be tested quickly and efficiently for their immuno-toxic potential.

The test may also be done by keeping a food diary, listing foods eaten and reactions noted, but that method is more time-consuming, and not as specific.

A person may be sensitive to a food, but not allergic, Food allergies or food sensitivities tax the immune system, trigger cravings of the very foods that we are allergic or sensitive to, and cause us to retain and put on more weight in the form of fat. Eating these foods puts us on a downward spiral towards illness, fatigue, psychological complaints, chronic disease, and more weight. The sensitivity causes toxic reactions in the body, causing cerebral problems, irritations, and serious illness.

If, after testing, a person is determined to have one or more food sensitivities, that particular food is eliminated from the diet, generally for two months. Some food may need to be permanently eliminated. Then a food rotation diet can be used.

GENETIC TESTING; 23ANDME; MTHFR; EPIGENETICS; EPIGENOMICS

Genetic testing uses laboratory methods to examine your genes, which are the DNA instructions inherited from both your parents. Genetic tests may be used to identify increased risks of health problems, to choose treatments, or to assess responses to treatments.

Genetic tests can help to:
- Diagnose disease
- Identify gene changes that are responsible for an already diagnosed disease
- Determine the severity of a disease
- Guide doctors in deciding on the best medicine or treatment to use for certain individuals
- Identify gene changes that may increase the risk to develop a disease
- Identify gene changes that could be passed on to children
- Screen newborn babies for certain treatable conditions

Genetic test results can be difficult to understand, however specialists like geneticists and genetic counselors can help explain what results might mean to you and your family. Because genetic testing gives you information about your DNA, which can be shared with other family members, sometimes a genetic test result may have implications for blood relatives of the person who was tested.

23andMe

23andMe uses cutting-edge technology to genotype DNA. The patient provides a saliva sample and mails the kit to the lab postage pre-paid. Results are returned via the internet. 23andMe is a FDA approved laboratory which meets quality standards for genotype testing.

MTHFR

Deficiency of the methylenetetrahydrofolate reductase (MTHFR) enzyme revealed in genetics testing increases risks of psychiatric disorders, neural tube defects, and high blood pressure during pregnancy, according to the National Institutes of Health.

The MTHFR enzyme plays a role in the conversion of homocysteine into methionine, the amino acids used by the body to make proteins and other compounds. MTHFR deficiency leads to increased levels of homocysteine in the bloodstream, while methionine levels decline. This results from the reduced ability of the body to process folate, which affects the brain and central nervous system.

The condition interferes with blood pressure, with increased effects among pregnant women. MTHFR deficiency can cause neural tube defects including spina bifida, a condition in which the bones of the spinal column fail to close completely during formation. Researchers also associate the MTHFR deficiency with stroke, cleft lip, heart diseases, breast cancer, and the glaucoma eye disorder. Like other diseases resulting from gene mutations, MTHFR deficiency shows large variations among those affected.

P.S. Both I and my step-grandson suffer from physical and central nervous system problems due to MTHFR.

Epigenomic; Epigenetic

According to the NIH, genetic and environmental factors can influence the body, resulting in problems like MTHFR deficiency. According to Dr. Mark Hyman and Dr. Steven Gundry genes are not rigid or concrete, but can be turned on or off by various environmental factors. Dr. Hyman states that what we eat is the leading environmental factor that most influences our genes. Healthy food will positively affect our genes. Unhealthy food will negatively affect our genes, leading to poor health.

HAIR ANALYSIS

Hair analysis can indicate the status of 21 minerals in the body and is an excellent overall health indicator. By examining the hair, exposure to lead, cadmium, mercury, arsenic, or other toxic pollutants can be determined. Hair permanently records the past events of one's trace element status. Concentrations in hair are often ten times greater than that of blood or urine. Hair more closely reflects body storage than does blood or urine, and will show toxicity when blood or urine will not. The alternative to hair analysis would be to do a biopsy on a body organ, which requires surgery, is expensive, and objectionable. Hair analysis is an excellent screening measurement and is simple, safe, and relatively inexpensive.

Only a small amount is needed for testing, and the hair is cut off where it will draw the least attention, usually from near the scalp or from the beard. This test is also painless. Atomic absorption spectrophotometry is used, whereby the hair is burned and minerals are measured by the light frequency given off while burning. In January 1985, a judge in the Federal District Court at Alexandria, VA, ruled that a multi-elemental spectral hair analysis is a useful guide in the hands of a health-care professional.

IRIDOLOGY

The theory and practice of Iridology asserts that parts of the iris reflect various areas of the body and the state of disease or health in those areas can be seen. The method states that the iris is divided into four zones and these zones are connected to various parts of the body by nerve fibers.

Iridology reveals the following health and personality traits:
- inherent predisposition toward health or disease
- inherent strengths and weaknesses
- strength of body constitution
- levels of health of organs and systems
- location of toxins and congestions
- nutritional deficiencies of vitamins and minerals
- chemical balance in the body
- basic personality traits
- introversion/extroversion tendencies
- right/left brain dominance
- relationship attractions/repulsions and why they're formed
- parent/child relationships
- gifts and talents

Certain eye colors have a predispoition to weakness of body systems. For example, blue eyes tend towards rheumatic, lymphatic, and tubercular weakness.

Iridology or iridiagnosis is the diagnosing of disease from spots appearing in the iris of the eye and originated with a Budapest physician, Ignatz Peczely, around 1880. Peczely stumbled onto the method in this fashion:

He captured an owl with a broken foot and noticed a black spot in the lower central region of the bird's iris. As the bird's bone healed, he observed a white ring developing around the black spot. Peczely theorized that the location of the spot represented the region of the broken foot and the spot represented scar tissue.

Dr. James Carter, who helped develop the soft contact lens, believes iridology works because the irises are intimately connected with the brain and the nervous system, as well as the circulatory system. Iris pigment, which is unusual because it has nerve endings, is constantly replaced as the eye color is maintained. Any abnormality in the body chemistry can disturb this process.

To utilize the science of iridology, the iris is examined using a 4X magnifying glass and a penlight. The texture, density, and pigmentation of the iris is observed. Acute signs of disease show up in the iris as lines, flakes, clouds, darkness, or spots. Using iridology as a diagnostic method can prevent certain factors from becoming full-blown disease. Looking into the eye and diagnosing according to this method is intricate and takes extensive training.

LIVE CELL ANALYSIS

Live cell analysis is a test which is done by pricking the fingertip and drawing a drop of blood from the finger onto a slide. The drop of blood is analyzed under a microscope at 100X, 400X, and 1000X magnification. This slide provides an instant, clear, and graphic picture of current health status and the need for any specific nutrients to support, strengthen, and rebuild weakened organs and systems.

Live cell analysis helps to identify present and potential problems:
- candida
- cholesterol
- liver problems
- poor circulation
- protoplast and s.p. progenitors that contribute to cancer, multiple sclerosis, and heart disease.
- uric acid crystals
- vitamin, mineral, and protein deficiency

Individual cells are the building blocks of life; they are vital to both the function and structure of all living things. The cell is in itself a living, functioning organism. The cell obtains its energy and maintains its life by utilizing oxygen and converting certain organic nutrients. If the cell is denied oxygen and nutrients due to a poor diet, stress, emotional upset, poor digestion, improper eating habits, toxic food, polluted water and air, then all these things will cause imbalance and cause the cell to degenerate.

Cells are formed in the body. Cells make up the tissues of the body. Organs are made up of this tissue. Live cell analysis allows us to see these changes on the cell level and identify the deficiency, as well as to determine organ function and problems.

The warning signs of cell deficiency are:

- depression and irritability
- headache
- loss of energy
- loss of sex drive
- memory lapses
- pre-mature aging
- tiredness and fatigue
- weight loss or gain

Live cell analysis, which had many years of research and case studies before becoming available to the public, can determine yeast in the body, food allergies, and any presence of infection—showing the ratio of red to white blood cells. This test can determine the effectiveness of oxygen reaching the tissues, fat intake, liver function, nutritional status, cholesterol, and triglyceride levels. Additionally platelets or red cell clumping, which forewarns of liver stress, can be detected. After treatment another live cell analysis is done to determine the effectiveness of treatment.

P.S. WHAT THE FUTURE MAY HOLD

My first encounter with Live Cell Analysis was when I took my son to a holistic practitioner and he was tested with this fairly new method. He had been sleeping a great deal, was tired a lot, and his grades were plummeting.

He acted like he was drugged, although he was not on drugs, and his personality had changed into something less than desirable.

The test results were very upsetting. A number of health problems were diagnosed. The good news is that his problem was resolved mainly with diet and specific supplements. I am happy to report that he has regained much of his health.

I talked to Susana Lombardi, founder of the We Care Health Center in California. She had heard from her physician that a disturbing trend is becoming apparent, based on a number of live cell analyses done. With each succeeding generation, the people seem to be less and less healthy, more and more tired. Senior citizens tested the best and children the worst.

I got to thinking about the kids at my son's school. They all looked healthy as he did, but what if they too, have severe health problems which affect learning, personality, and social behavior? Are we so addicted to fast foods, candy, soda pop, and other junk food that we are changing the health and course of our civilization?

THERMOGRAPHY

Thermography is a non-invasive, painless measurement of blood flow and circulation through recording the infrared emission of heat from the body. Thermography records skin temperature photographically.

A thermograph is a heat photograph which looks something like a negative in that the tones are reversed. Pictures can also be taken in color. The coldest areas (less circulation) show up as black or blue, and the warmest as orange or red. The principle behind thermography is that inflammation in the body radiates extra heat to the skin surface which can be picked up by an infrared detector.

This ability to measure circulation proves invaluable in diagnosing and treating physical problems. Strokes, potential arteriosclerosis of the hands and feet, and gangrene are some circulatory illnesses which can be detected.

More heat emanates from tumors than from normal tissue. This sophisticated machine renders the most minute temperature variations and heat emissions as multi-colored patterns. Thermography can be performed to detect tumors and to study the breast to help reveal breast disease and cancer, even before a lump can be found.

Hospitals, clinics and doctors are using this method to diagnose such ailments as arthritis, back pains, and even headaches. Dr. Paul Ruegsegger, a New York internist specializing in headache detection and treatment, says he has employed thermography with great success.

ULTRASOUND TESTING

High frequency sound waves are different from light waves and can be used in medical diagnosing. Sound waves pass through the skin, tissue, and organs. Thus, a doctor can choose the tissue she wishes to image by changing the frequency of the sound wave.

The information projected by the sound wave is recorded by moving the patient or the transducer to sense the inner tissue. Using ultrasound as a diagnostic tool is also called sonography or sonar, and is based on echoes. With ultrasound, a transducer is placed on the patient and produces a sound wave that bounces and is recorded on a TV screen. Sometimes a 3-D image can be viewed.

Ultrasound is painless, invisible, and cannot be heard by the human ear. It produces images like X-rays but can differentiate between the different tissues. Done routinely it poses no medical risk.

Echocardiography, based on ultrasound, uses sound waves to create a picture of the heart and to illuminate the smallest of blood vessels. Cardiologist Steven Feinstein, MD, University of Chicago Medical Center, fills a sugar solution with a fine cloud of air bubbles, which, when injected, reflect the sound waves. Doctors can watch blood flow on a television screen in places they could never see before. Ultrasound as a testing device can detect and delineate disease in the following areas:

- Cardiology—detecting congenital or acquired heart disease
- Obstetrics—determining stage of pregnancy and for fetal visualization
- Abdominal examinations—gallbladder, liver, urinary tract, bladder, prostate, and kidneys
- Determining circulatory disease
- Mammography—determining breast health
- Determining if a cancerous tumor is malignant

CONCLUSION

As I've mentioned, my reason for creating this book has been intensely personal. For most of my life I've been sickly and unhappy, which kept me out of school and being able to play as a child, and, as an adult, hardly able to be satisfactorily employed nor healthfully parent my children. I received traditional medical care for years without much difference.

Before my first visit to a holistic physician, I filled out an in-depth four-page questionnaire of my symptoms and history. Then I had a two-hour consultation with Dr. Kwiker. After questioning me thoroughly, he commented, "Wow! You are really sick!" I was 32 years old. I broke down and cried. Finally, someone was listening.

A new world opened up for me.

Impressed and eager, I began to search for other alternative methods that might help my health improve even more. I've personally experienced approximately 95% of the methodologies I've compiled in this book.

My overall health has improved significantly and at 70 I'm healthier than I've been in decades. Health, I've discovered, is a life-long process. I consider health a verb, a journey, and a process, rather than a destination. In that regard health is ever-expanding. One can never have too much health.

Alternatives for Everyone is not simply about my own struggle and success. I'm hoping to pass on valuable information to you and your loved ones. My job, as I see it, is to simply gather all the methods I know into one volume to assist in your search, to give you a starting place.

If you have been sick, in pain, or suffering, and can't seem to get better, don't give up. Keep looking. *Alternatives for Everyone, a Guide to Non-Tra-*

ditional Health Care 2nd edition is written for you, for your health concerns, and to share non-traditional methods outside of mainstream medicine.

If you have problems, there is an underlying cause— and perhaps a cure as well. There are alternatives for everyone.

I've recently created a website as a continuation of this book. The website contains links for further research.

https://thymelauren.wixsite.com/thymely-one/alternative-health-links

Best of health to you!
Lauren O. Thyme   July 13, 2017

thyme.lauren@gmail.com
https://www.facebook.com/lauren.thyme

www.ingramcontent.com/pod-product-compliance
Lightning Source LLC
Chambersburg PA
CBHW060851280326
41934CB00007B/1009